To Darren

Love,

Shayla Rose

April 29, 2019

Stuck on the Sidelines

The Reality of Facing
Postural Orthostatic Tachycardia Syndrome

Shayla Rose

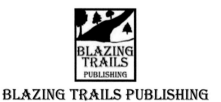

BLAZING TRAILS PUBLISHING

Library of Congress Control Number: 2019937225

ISBN: 978-1-7336845-0-7

This book is recounted based on my personal memory, although names of people, places, or occupations referenced in this book may have been changed for privacy reasons.

Published by Blazing Trails Publishing
Boston, MA
blazingtrailspublishing@aol.com

Printed in the United States of America
First Edition April 2019

DEDICATION

This book is for you, yes you — the one with the heavy heart
I know that you're worried, you've had a rough start
I wrote this for you — for the ones alone
For the ones in the hospital and the ones at home
For the ones in bed who cannot walk
For the ones who are too sick to talk
For the ones who are crying in fear
For the ones who have no more tears
For the ones who are caught in self-blame
For the ones whose illness has caused them much shame
I know dysautonomia from the inside
I can feel its impact, from that I can't hide
It's invisible, even though it's very real to me
The symptoms nobody else can see
I know what it looks like — I can see its face
It can be every age and every race
I know what it sounds like — I've heard it before
It's the voices of millions, it's a silenced roar

— "Stuck on the Sidelines" by Shayla Rose

I dedicate this book to everyone who has been affected by dysautonomia, for those we have lost, and for those who continue fighting.

Your illness may be invisible, but you are not. We are in this fight together, hand in hand, and we will not give up.
Awareness lies in you, let your voice be heard.

CONTENTS

INTRODUCTION

I HAD A REALIZATION when I was eighteen. Behind sets of blinds, through foggy window panes and on the other side of closed doors, there were others who endured the same symptoms and faced the same battles as me. There were millions of other people who were also sidelined from society. I was never the only one, even though it always seemed that way. It was in that moment of quiet realization that I began to write this book, hoping to finally let my voice—and the silenced voices of countless others—be heard.

I grew up as a healthy kid. Chronic illness never once scratched the surface of my young mind. I was energetic, full of wonder, and always eager for adventure. As a child, I was under the impression that illness was temporary. I never knew that there were illnesses that existed where people didn't get better. I thought that the key to good health and longevity was exercise and healthy food choices. I never knew that an illness could lay dormant for years within us, without us even knowing.

My plummet to the sidelines was slow in the making, I didn't see it coming. Although there were small signs along the way, hinting to my impending decline, myself and those around me were generally heedless to them.

My first memory of feeling different was when I was ten years old. I was attending my friend's birthday sleepover, and after a long sleepless night, I awoke the next morning feeling indescribably different. I felt like I was still dreaming, even though I was awake. I didn't know it at the time, but I was experiencing a sensation known as depersonalization, and I was terrified. Nobody around me took my symptoms seriously. That afternoon I cried myself to sleep on my living room floor. Luckily, when I awoke hours later, this symptom became nothing more than a taunting memory I hoped to never relive.

Throughout the next couple years, more strange things were happening to me. I began to develop random episodes of what I learned to call "whiplash" — which I would later learn was neck-tongue syndrome. If I turned my head too quickly, a paralyzing pain would shoot up my neck, my tongue would turn numb and my vision would fade to black. Then, as quickly as it came, this crippling event would leave. I never mentioned this to anyone, because at the time I thought this was something everyone experienced.

As time went on, I began to black out nearly every time I stood up. I was told to hydrate more — but it didn't help. When I was twelve years old, I was constantly feeling out of breath and was diagnosed with a "touch of asthma". The inhaler I was prescribed did little to help my symptoms, so eventually I stopped using it altogether and accepted my breathlessness.

I was at a confused place in my life. After trying to warn others of my infrequent symptoms, and getting virtually nowhere each time, I began to suppress my own worries and learned to live with my strange symptoms for as long as I possibly could. Eventually, just a few short months later, the harsh reality that my odd symptoms were leading me to finally hit.

I soon would become a different person — virtually overnight — and I never would be the same. My childhood was about to crumble away right before my eyes, and my body was about to become an enemy who disowned me from the inside out.

Postural Orthostatic Tachycardia Syndrome (POTS) is the most common form of dysautonomia. Despite affecting so much of our population (both young and old), most people have never heard of POTS. Imagine being sidelined from society by symptoms no test can detect, and no other person can see?

It wasn't easy to decide to share my personal story. Combing through all the layers of my journey produced a reel of emotions, ones that I buried over time. But I owe it to myself, and to others who have derailed down the lonely, frightening, and uncomfortable path through chronic illness, to show first-hand the life of a dysautonomia patient. It is my hope that my years of sickness do not go wasted, and that by reading my story, more people understand how life-altering and disabling dysautonomia really is. Welcome to my chronic illness story.

Chapter One
The Beginning of the End

One day you feel so fine, you just don't think of pain
One day it is so sunny, you just don't think of rain
One day you can see the landscape and admire all the shades
The next day all your precious sight fades
One day you can walk, and you can even run
The next day you cannot stand, your legs each weigh a ton
It is so important to savor each day
To use your given strengths and live life all the way

— *"Live Life all the Way" by Shayla Rose*

AFTER A LONG summer break, filled with carefree days under the warm New England sunshine, a new school year was about to begin. Like most kids, I hated to say goodbye to the long, homework-free days of summer vacation. Getting letters in the mail announcing my new teachers made the upcoming school year even more real. I savored every minute that was left of summer, until there were no more minutes remaining.

My back leaned against the cool white refrigerator—as it did on every first day of school.

"Say cheese!" my mom said with a smile, her index finger on the shutter button of her famous Kodak camera.

I formed my lips into a smile, and I stood up straight and proud in my new school clothes. Butterflies fluttered through my stomach in anxious waves as my mom took a photo of my brother and I—hoping to preserve each defying moment.

1

"I love you, be careful! I will see you when you get home, okay?" my mom said to me as she zipped up my backpack and reached for a hug.

"Do you have everything?" she asked once more.

"Yes. I love you," I replied as I looked into her eyes and walked out the front door, blowing kisses.

Today was the first day of seventh grade, and the next few weeks would be a transitional time for me, in more ways than one.

I stood at the end of our driveway alongside my older brother as we waited for the school bus to arrive. Soon the high-pitched whistle of the school buses brakes entered my young ears. The long yellow school bus stopped at the end of the driveway and our familiar bus driver welcomed us on.

"Hey guys, how are you?" she asked us excitedly through her thick Boston accent.

"Hi! I'm doing good," I replied as I searched for a place to sit down.

I looked left and right as I walked down the skinny aisle, placing my hand on top of each grey leather seat. I had never seen the bus so packed before. It seemed that nearly every seat was occupied. I had hoped to sit alongside my friend during the journey into seventh grade, but there was simply no room. Her stop was before mine and her desperate attempts to save me a seat were unsuccessful. We exchanged a worried expression before I ultimately sat with a much older stranger in the back of the bus.

After an uncomfortable bus ride, I stood inside of the junior high school among a crowd of others. The hallways were filled with monotone noise. A mixture of laughter, screams and nerves jittered the building. My palms dripped sweat and my legs shook inside my new jeans. My new shoes squeaked with every step, providing good traction upon the waxed tile. Finally, after a long search, I landed precisely where my wrinkled paper schedule said I should be.

The classroom was already full, it looked like I was nearly late. I sat down in one of the few desks that were empty and dropped my purple backpack to the floor with an appropriate thump. I turned to my right, and spotted an old friend sitting in the row of desks beside mine.

"Hey!" I muttered, hoping to rekindle an old friendship.

She looked at me and scoffed, before turning away and talking to her other friends.

I felt rejected by her rude response, and immediately regretted being so friendly.

In front of me sat a girl with red hair. I had never seen her before, but she continually turned around and looked at me. Eventually, during one of her predictable head turns, I decided to speak to her.

"Hello!" I said politely.

She creased her brow and quickly faced forward.

Wow, I wonder what I did wrong?

Seventh grade hadn't officially started yet, and I was already feeling very uncomfortable. For the first time I felt alone in a crowd of familiar faces. I wasn't sure what the summer had done to my classmates, but most girls were now wearing makeup, and most boys grew a foot taller and spoke like men. I was stuck in a whirlwind of puberty and somehow lost the memo explaining the do's and don'ts. Apparently, by the reaction from those around me, I was already starting off on the wrong foot. I had nothing to do but to remain quiet, seeking refuge in my thoughts.

The days continued as I began to adjust to the new school year. Luckily, not all my classmates were unaccepting, and I began to really enjoy some of my classes.

Independence was being introduced into our lives more than it ever had been before. We were on our own, no more single file lines, or sharing coat closets. Seventh grade was different, and I was adapting. But, seventh grade wasn't all I would be forced to adapt to. As the weather grew hotter, my body struggled to function. It was becoming clear that the summer heat was not yet ready to succumb to autumns crisp air. Even though it was early September, we were in the middle of a long heatwave.

As I sat at my desk in math class, my heart seemed to beat too fast. My thirst increased as I flirted with passing out. Despite my odd symptoms, I was too shy to let my ailments be known. My teachers and classmates were just as overheated as I was, so I didn't want to complain.

The classrooms were sweltering inside of the un-air-conditioned school. Everyone tried desperately to seek relief by opening windows, dimming the lights, and setting up floor fans. But despite their efforts, the classrooms were still stuffy and sweaty.

Every day more people excused themselves to fill up water bottles or go to the nurse's office. Each day I sat in the front row of class overcome by dizziness and heat. Soon I struggled to see the giant smart board ten feet in front of me, each equation morphed into a fuzzy blur.

As I dismounted the school bus each afternoon, my driveway seemed to grow longer. My legs and body couldn't keep up. The after-school snacks I devoured seemed to supply less and

4

less energy with each passing day. I dragged myself through every mundane task as my energy reserves slowly became depleted. Before long, the only task I could accomplish after school was a long rest on the couch.

My mom grew concerned as I told her about my recent visual changes. So, one evening after school, my mom brought me to the eye doctor. I explained to my optometrist how I struggled to see the smart board at school. I told him how everything blurred into an illegible line and I often felt lightheaded. He looked at my eyes closely before sending me on my way home with flying colors. I walked through the parking lot with large sunglasses covering my eyes, serving as a protective shield for my dilated pupils. I sat in the car and rode home, giddy that I had good vision, perplexed at why I felt so indescribably different.

Several days later I laid on the gym floor at school, surrounded by dozens of others.

"Ten sit-ups!" my gym coach called out stretch after stretch, as he prowled around to correct the stragglers.

I was so weak and exhausted that soon I just laid there motionless and defeated. The stretches, crunches and push-ups seemed so much harder than they once used to, and my body simply couldn't take anymore. I laid on the gym floor as still as a stone, waiting for the gym coach to make eye contact with me so that I could swiftly regain my pose, as if I had never stopped in the first place. I was the biggest straggler who was never caught.

"Okay!" the gym coach shouted.

Just as the word left his lips the entire class quickly started across the gym. Somehow, I missed out on the coach's important announcement and I was left lying on the gym floor alone. I looked to my far right where a glimmer of sunshine illuminated the waxed gym floors. I followed the light up and saw a stampede of gym sneakers. Quickly, I ran to them.

"Where are we going?" I asked the crowd repetitively to no avail.

My class and I walked out the heavy gym doors and into the early morning sunshine and dewy grass. I followed my classmates as we walked to a nearby field and ran the perimeter. I found the exercise pointless and unnecessarily exhausting. My heavy feeling of lightheadedness was creeping back on me. I felt like I was in a fog of impending doom, as if at any moment my body would collapse, and I would wake up to my gym teacher hovered over me. Somehow, I escaped this nightmarish thought that passed through my mind daily.

The laps seemed to never end, each one I thought was the last, but ten more seemed to remain.

"C'mon Shayla! Pick up those feet!" my gym coach yelled at me.

I began to ignore the calls being made to me to keep running. I walked slower than a turtle and immersed inside myself listening to my revving body. My head pounded, my vision pulsated, my legs were rubberized, and my hands were soaked. I was certain one more step would kill me. But it didn't.

I came home that day to a bouquet of colorful daisies.

"Happy thirteenth birthday!" my mother shouted as I stepped over the threshold and into the kitchen.

I greeted her with a grin before accepting my flowers, which served as a welcome gift to adolescence. We talked briefly about the independence and significance of entering my teenage years before I sat down for an after-school snack and relief to my indescribable sensations.

My future held a giant secret that would soon be revealed. What was about to happen would change the course of my adolescence forever.

Chapter Two
Captive by a Border of Roses

My mind is so cloudy, I cannot think
It feels like my boat is starting to sink
I was once so strong, and I could do so much
But the elements have left me out of touch
I could support the weight on my shoulders
I walked over pebbles that were once boulders
But it crept up on me, as it laid dormant in the dark
It came to haunt me, and burn out my spark

— *"Sinking" by Shayla Rose*

IT WAS ON an early September morning when my life completely changed.

My mother's voice echoed down the hallway and into my delicate ears.

"Wake up Shayla!" she hollered.

My eye lids parted and then closed again.

"Shayla! C'mon, it's time for school!"

I opened my eyes and gazed around my bedroom. A deep sense of transparency laid within me—I felt so far away from life. I felt like I was in a dream even though I was awake. It was as though I was stuck somewhere in between, riding the divide of the conscious world and the unconscious one. The same distant feeling that overcame me on the day of that infamous sleepover a couple years prior had now returned.

My entire body was coated in a heavy blanket of fatigue. Each limb felt like a weighted sandbag. I could hardly catch my breath—I had no air to spare. My clouded mind was as fatigued as the rest of my body. I had no words, and no thoughts.

I had long since missed the school bus and my mom was now hovered over my bedside begging for answers to my unmotivated body.

"You don't feel good?" she asked me.

I looked deep into her blue eyes—hoping they would somehow take all the confusion and symptoms away from me—but they didn't. I felt like I was floating in an altered reality—everything seemed so unreal. I closed my eyes and searched deep within myself for an answer. Desperately I tried to find the right words to convey how I was feeling.

"I'm…dizzy…" I claimed with a breathless stutter, cringing at the volume of my own voice.

My body was so weak, and my mind was spent. It occurred to me with great sureness, I had reached my breaking point.

The breaking point I had now reached was coming for some time. My body had been falling apart for a while before this odd September morning, but few could see it. Even my pediatrician—who I had seen recently for my odd symptoms—couldn't fully understand the complexity of how I had been feeling.

They thought I was coming down with a cold. My parents and pediatrician had hoped that my strange downward spiral was simply the beginning of a virus—something that would ravage my body for a mere week before fading away. I shared their hope, but at the same time, I didn't believe it.

I became a seventh grader who was stranded in bed, having exhaustion that required much more sleep than a twenty-four-hour day could provide. My body was weak and unsteady, making walking or standing nearly impossible. I was now nothing more than a hollowed-out version of who I used to be.

Going to the bathroom became the most daunting task I could envision. The bathroom was only about ten feet away from my bedroom, but to me it seemed so much farther. I dreaded the task, and tried so hard to avoid it, but mother nature could only be ignored for so long. Soon, with my mother's help and steadiness, my daunting bathroom trip would be completed, and I would be back in the comfort of my bed, having to sleep even longer to recover from the excursion.

I felt like I was fading away. My all-too-familiar bedroom now scared me—it didn't look the same. I felt so distant from life, and no matter how hard I tried, I could not escape the clouded sensation of feeling as though I was in a constant dream.

As my days of being bedridden continued, my concern grew, and my hope faded. I struggled to understand what I did wrong. What caused my body to suddenly just fall apart? I clung to the hope that it would get better—that the mysterious virus would soon lift away—but the passing days continued to show me no mercy.

I watched my ceiling fan spin effortlessly above me in repetitive circles. I watched the trees outside sway back and forth in the late summers breeze, only hoping to someday sit beneath their shade once more. I stared at the old photograph of my third-grade soccer team and wondered if I would ever again have the strength to kick a goal.

I counted each rose in the border that encircled my bedroom several times each day. The number I studied so deeply. Fifty-two—there were fifty-two roses.

It was becoming very apparent to us all that whatever was plaguing me was not the virus or cold that we all hoped it was. As I sat in the waiting room of my pediatrician's office, tears dripped down my cheeks. I held tightly on to my father's arm, terrified. Each second of sitting upright felt like an eternity of agonizing vertigo and impending syncope. I struggled to function away from my bed. My eye lids closed in an uncomfortable darkness, proving to be the only shield I had against my taunting reality.

The waiting soon ended, and I was directed into a small room with white walls and neutral colored paintings. My eyes couldn't stay open longer than a few seconds. I felt like I had boulders on each lid, making it impossible to stay awake. I sat on the exam table slowly before lying down and resting my head on the paper covered pillow. Each movement of my body made an obnoxiously loud crinkle, which only spooked me more.

"I don't feel good," I quietly said to my parents, whimpering.

My mom stood up and stroked my leg with her hand. Behind her sat my father, who wore a face of concern.

The doorknob slowly turned, followed by a subtle knock. My pediatrician entered the small exam room and greeted my parents and I before she sat down on a swiveling black stool. She placed her laptop on the cramped grey counter and began to ask me and my parents questions. After listening to my peculiar symptoms, the doctor stood up and began to examine me.

She shined a light at my eyes, a black cuff squeezed my arm, a stethoscope listened to my heart. Her cold hands put pressure on either side of my lymph nodes. Soon, she sat back down on her stool and turned towards my parents.

She muttered few words, "I'm not sure why she feels this way. I mean, everything looks normal."

"What about Lyme disease?" my mother asked.

The doctor shook her head no. She felt that the possibility of me having Lyme disease was slim, and in her mind, was not worth investigating further.

My hope was weaved in one tense cable that supported me above the ominous sea below. The cable was severed by my doctor's hopeless truth. It was as if the words my doctor spoke were only confirming my depressive thoughts. Nobody knew why I was suddenly so sick, but I knew I wasn't going to get better without finding a cause to my sudden, debilitating symptoms.

My eyes produced pails of tears. I was inconsolable and could not hold onto the intense emotions any longer. My body didn't feel right, and my doctor couldn't tell me why. My heart and hopes shattered—I was just as alone as I thought I was.

My pediatrician watched me break apart in tears. She attempted to reassure me as she stood up and placed her hand on my shaking shoulder.

"You will get better, I promise," she whispered.

The words that filled my ears did little to comfort my torn soul, they only brushed the surface of my raw, deep-rooted emotions. I felt that her promise was a cop-out, a distant hope that wouldn't be reached.

I drowned in tears on the ride home. My cheeks were drenched, and my eyelashes could have been wrung out like a towel. My bottom lip quivered, my chin twitched, and my head pounded in overwhelming emotion.

I looked through my waterlogged vision and saw an equally as sorrow-filled sky. The rain poured down in tear drops, the sky was filled with ominous and hopeless grey clouds. I felt like my life was ending, from the inside out. Each worsening symptom seemed to bring me one step closer to the edge. I felt alone in my suffering. Nobody else could comprehend how I felt.

"We aren't giving up," my dad told me in part.

As we drove through the rainstorm, I found my God-given rainbows. My parents had the ability to offer me reassurance in the darkest of times. With every mile my tears evaporated, and my whimpers faded.

My old self—the girl with infectious laughter and vibrant energy was gone. She was stolen in the shadow of a September night and there were no signs of her ever coming back.

Chapter Three
A Day, a Week, a Month

Without darkness we underappreciate the light
Without blindness we never realize the importance of sight
Without someone's absence, we can't cherish their presence
The truth of the matter is, everything can change in mere seconds
Time, it evolves us all, it is the routine of our existence
After all, tomorrow would never come without time's assistance
It's the inevitable, for things to stop on a dime
But until it is taken, we don't appreciate time

— *"Time" by Shayla Rose*

TIME—IT TAUNTED ME. I had never felt the impact of it this much before. I watched the clock on the nearby wall every day. I simply was waiting and watching—waiting for the time when my life would go back to normal, watching for my lost time to be replaced. But neither happened. Time served as a constant reminder of what was, and what wasn't. The world around me continued as it always had before. I couldn't grasp this phenomenon.

I had been ill for nearly a month now, and my quality of life was unchanging in its demise. I had suffered a terrible loss of myself, and another day of grueling symptoms seemed pointless and frightening.

I was still bedridden, but I now spent my days downstairs in our living room. My parents set up a cot for me, which served as my daybed. I was hesitant at first—to leave the comfort of my bed upstairs—but ultimately, I was happy with their decision.

I was dizzy twenty-four seven and became dependent on others for every task. I went from a thirteen-year-old with boundless energy, to a thirteen-year-old brushing her teeth over a bowl and taking a shower on a stool.

As time continued to tick, and no answers were yet found, my frustration mounted. I was beyond fatigued, both emotionally and physically. I was beaten down by my new life—one that I didn't choose. I was scared by the unknown and frustrated that I couldn't find help.

The further I investigated my symptoms the more confused I became. I couldn't stand up for long, and I could hardly walk. I couldn't hold a conversation without closing my eyes. My heart raced and skipped. I was out of breath, heat intolerant, I struggled to swallow, and I even sometimes struggled to eat.

I remember the dialogue as if it were yesterday. I was lying on my daybed on one late afternoon, wrapped in blankets and whimpering in heavy lightheadedness and detachment. My eyes were closed, my brain was half-asleep. My brother entered the room, I could tell it was him simply by the way his foot struck the squeaky board in our living room hallway. He sat on the couch nearby and asked my mother ever so causally,

"Is Shayla going to die?"

The words haunted me, in fact, they still do. Perhaps the haunting part goes further than the innocent words them self, because I did not know the answer—nobody did.

Am I going to die?

Nobody could shed light on my most important questions. Nobody knew the answers. I could sense the unsureness in my mother's voice as she responded to him.

"Well I hope not!" she replied.

My symptoms were so debilitating, that I felt like I was dying. Inside my body was at war with itself. Nothing seemed to be functioning right—my entire system was misfiring.

By this point I had looked into the eyes belonging to doctors of many interests, and yet even still, I had no explanation for my faltering health.

I visited a neurologist at a private practice. The small practice before me resembled a house more than a medical building. I looked around and absorbed every detail of the practice, from the outdated wallpapered walls to the carpeted floors, every inch of the doctor's office was old. Most patients stood or leaned against the wall, there were not enough chairs to hold everyone. As my eyes scanned along the wall of strangers, I noticed that they all had the same washed face of boredom and annoyance. It was clear that they had been waiting a while.

The receptionist was tense and overwhelmed, her interactions with us and other patients was quick and snippy. It was fair to say that she had her hands full. She was overwhelmed by the amount of work in front of her, and, being the only receptionist there, her break was likely overdue.

After waiting for what seemed to be forever, I was called into a small room for my vitals to be taken. But as I sat down, and gazed at the floor, my heart sunk in embarrassment.

Suddenly I realized I was wearing my old, battered sneakers. My sneakers had rips and holes in them, and I couldn't believe I had accidentally worn them out of the house. They were so dirty and old. To most they were just sneakers, but to me they were a reminder of my once-functional life. My sneakers had walked me through so many fun summer days, from gripping the pedals on my bicycle, to grasping the slippery rocks on our early morning fishing trips. My sneakers were there for all my active adventures. These sneakers were a shrine—one of the last reminders left from my healthy life.

Soon, I was sitting across from my new doctor who sat at a shiny wooden desk. He had an unusual appearance for a doctor. He was a very large man, nearly as wide as he was tall. He had frizzy red hair, and a thick accent. He was dressed in a suit and didn't even carry a stethoscope. I felt like I was in the bank, facing the manager for a loan that was overdue.

He asked my parents and I many questions about my illness before having me sit on an exam table located on the opposite side of his office. He checked my reflexes and my eyes before retreating to his desk and sitting in his large, molded chair.

He presumed my illness was caused by migraines. My mother had a history of migraines, and he felt that the symptoms I was experiencing was my body's way of replicating them. He prescribed me topiramate, a medication aimed at combating my dizziness, or, at least that was the plan.

After trying the topiramate for a brief time, my memory faded, and my arms, legs, feet, and hands turned into a constant feeling of tingling and numbness. The medication did not help my underlying symptoms and seemed to only make things worse. We went back to this doctor, but he soon released me from his care.

We continued to search—search for whatever it was that was causing my downward spiral. We were all looking tirelessly for a cure—a cure for something we couldn't name.

I was referred to a pediatric cardiologist, who had a satellite office close to our local hospital. He was a middle-aged man with a wiry brown beard that was beginning to give way to grey.

He was very thorough in his examination. He listened to my heart closely, as though it held a secret clue in every beat. The stethoscope stayed on my chest for what seemed like several minutes as he listened intently. I stared off at the floor and wondered what my heart was possibly telling him. A young woman soon came in and took over the stethoscope. I watched her become mesmerized by my heartbeat as though it was the latest hit on the radio.

After a lengthy session of listening to my internal drum, the cardiologist dropped words I had never heard of before, 'mitral valve prolapse' and 'orthostatic intolerance' were two of the words that were highlighted in our conversation. These words meant nothing to me though, as I had never heard of them before.

The doctor assured me that my heart was healthy. He wrote me a prescription for fludrocortisone, a medication aimed at helping the body better retain salt, which in turn raises blood pressure and combats tachycardia. It was his hope that this medication would alleviate my symptoms.

I visited this cardiologist multiple times thereafter. The medication he prescribed did little to help my symptoms, and eventually I stopped taking it altogether. The doctor never did have an explanation for me. He didn't know why I was experiencing so many symptoms, and quite frankly, he stopped believing me. Eventually, he too, didn't have the answers.

With so many strange symptoms revoking the life within me, my parents took me to the hospital emergency room several times during my worst of flares. My parents always wore the same washed face of worry as we entered the emergency room doors.

We always went in hoping that today would be the day that we would find all the answers—today would be the end of the nightmare. We hoped that some doctor would come in and fine tune my body so that I could be better again, but this was merely a distant hope.

Every doctor I saw muttered the same ruthless truth. They could not help me. They did not know what was wrong with me.

"Everything looks fine," they told me again and again.

Each time, I was discharged without a diagnosis. Left to float back into society with tears in my eyes. I felt like I was dying, but my doctors were sure I wasn't. They did not know what was wrong though, and, at thirteen years old, not knowing was an answer I was forced to swallow.

"You seem healthy," they would say, as they looked directly into my tired eyes, watched me sway side to side on the exam table and black out on my way out their office door.

"Your tests all came back good, you're healthy!" they would tell me, as though it was a cause for celebration.

I always looked down at the floor in defeat. I was glad that my tests came back good, but at the same time my high achieving test results seemed to only clothe me in a layer of confusion and regret. My results never reflected how lousy I felt, and I often wondered why my body couldn't be more truthful. I couldn't understand it, I felt like I was dying on the inside, yet my body looked fine on the outside. I was imploding from a sickness no test could detect, and no other human could see. Soon, the invisibility of my illness became even more frustrating.

"You should see a psychologist," doctors began to suggest, implying that my symptoms were nothing more than a self-imposed mental trap of anxiety.

I was a small voice each professional was able to silence, I was a complicated case that no doctor made the time for. I faced a reality I could not escape and longed for freedom from my illness. I felt invalidated in the offices of supposed superheroes in lab coats. I felt transparent in a world of opacity.

What if it is all in my head? What if I, somehow, caused all of this?

I became poisoned by their words, by their uneducated, silence-seeking diagnoses. I began to not only believe them, but I began to downplay how I felt. Inside I fought a finger pointing war of self-blame.

I used to think that doctors could cure anything. It wasn't until I became chronically ill that I realized, doctors only know as much as the medical books they read and the patients they've treated. I didn't fall into the categories that most other patients did. I was a unique case.

Chapter Four
It's All in Your Head

I'm on my knees pleading
Inside I am grieving
I'm running a race but every meter I fall
I try to stand up, but my pride is so small
The life I now lead is so different from before
My entire self has changed, from my body to my core
I try to keep up, but my body isn't strong
They all say I'm fine, but I know something is wrong
I don't care what they have to say
Their words and education don't make me okay

— *"Pleading" by Shayla Rose*

I SAT IN THE OFFICE of a psychologist and wiped my cold, sweaty palms on my jeans. I placed my water bottle between my thighs and looked to my mother for reassurance. My mom was there to support me and to be the stereo surround sound when I needed my opinions reinforced. The psychologist, Dr. Stein, sat across from me, only a wooden desk and our own opinions separated us.

"So, tell me about what's going on," Dr. Stein said candidly.

Our conversation started out frank and polite. Just the truth. I laid out my reality and the whirlwind of symptoms I had encountered within the past couple months to this woman behind the desk. But the reaction I received was not expected, and before I knew it, I was in the hot seat—feeling ashamed of myself for reasons far beyond my control.

"Why don't you want to go to school?" she asked me.

"Because I am dizzy," I respectfully pointed out the obvious.

"What does dizzy feel like?"

"Like I'm in a dream..."

Dr. Stein looked at me as though she was craving more, but I couldn't elaborate. The words would not form. My mind drew a blank.

What does dizzy feel like?

I began to question my very own authenticity.

Dr. Stein continued her questions, "Why can't you go to school though?"

"Because I am dizzy. I can't walk around the school, I'm sick. I have to take a shower at like one or two in the afternoon because I get so bad. I have to rest a lot."

"Yeah, but what time does school get out?"

"...Two o'clock..."

"So why can't you try to go to school?"

Dr. Stein stared at my mother with a puzzled look. My heart sank, my soul shattered, my fists clenched, and my mind raced. I looked at my mom, hoping to find reassurance, but none was offered. The rest of the appointment I shut my ears. In my mind this psychologist didn't matter anymore.

This was the first of many times I would be left with a choice to either sit down and take the criticism or pull my courage out of my back pocket and stand up for myself. Ultimately, I chose the former. I felt so lifeless, and this woman was not worth the energy of offering an explanation to. It seemed that every response I gave was questioned. I simply could not win.

After exchanging our opinions, I realized that Dr. Stein was not there to help me cope with the overwhelming feeling of grief I felt for losing my healthy self. She was not there to help me understand that it was okay to feel sick, to feel left out, or hopeless. She was there for one reason only—to cure me of my fake, self-inflicted illness and send me back to school. She treated me as if I was the cause of my own demise—as if the enemy I had been trying so desperately to name existed only in my mirrored reflection.

At a time when I needed help off the bewildered road of chronic illness, I was given a swift, invalidating push back down. But I would get up. Someday.

What followed was frustration and defeat. Days, weeks, and months of depressive thoughts and self-blame.

What if she's right? Can I go back to school?

I laid on my left side, encased with sheets and preparing for yet another nap. The grandmother clock in the neighboring kitchen chimed three times. It was the afternoon as I envisioned my classmates spilling out of the junior high school. Every day, from my warm bed, I would count down each second awaiting the school bell, just as I had once before.

My phone beside me soon beeped. I turned over with a sigh. It was another text message from a classmate, telling me of the latest school event I seemed to miss. My heart sank every time I reached for my phone.

Why do I have to miss everything?

"How r u doing?", "Wen will u b back?", "We miss u", the texts continued.

Some may think these text messages would be comforting, but they weren't. Although I was thankful for the one or two classmates who did not forget me, hearing from them served only as a reminder of what I was missing. It was as if I patched my wounded heart with a Band-Aid, and every text message only ripped the Band-Aid off, exposing my bleeding heart beneath.

"Wht do u have?" my friend asked me, "Do u think u can come back nxt wk?"

I could not respond. My symptoms were not attributed to any obvious cause. The more these questions were asked, the more alone and afraid I felt. These questions presented me with my terrifying reality. I was suffering from an undiagnosed illness. How could I know my prognosis without a diagnosis?

Each ding of my phone seemed to push me one inch closer to the edge of a cliff. My thoughts raced.

I am alone, I am undiagnosed, I am giving up.

Each day I laid there, covered in cool sheets and fearing my symptoms. I experienced a terrible set of ailments that never went away. Consistently I felt as if I were dreaming, as if I was detached from the world around me, only being a bystander of life. Each time the dog barked, or a dish was dropped, I felt like I lost my grip—as if these unexpected noises interrupted my ability to hold on to reality for several seconds.

Aside from my frightening detachment, I became a host to other symptoms, including lightheadedness, weak legs that were barely strong enough to support me, adrenaline surges, tingling feet and hands, noise sensitivity, light sensitivity, difficulty swallowing, inability to feel certain parts of my body, brain fog, fatigue and more. As my illness progressed, I soon developed a new tick of unintentional eye rolling. Perhaps this newly found, uncontrollable quirk was a bi-product from the stress of my undiagnosed illness.

As I laid on the cot's old springy mattress, I sat and wondered.

How will I face the world from this position, from this cot older than myself? Will I forever be forgotten, remembered only as the girl who used to be, and not the girl that is? Will my illness continue to define me, or will I soon define it?

I trudged through these lingering questions daily, only filling the unanswered void with distractions rather than solid answers.

As if the suffocating weight of my illness was not enough, a letter soon arrived in the mail. My absences from the junior high school were accumulating.

I would be lying if I said that this letter came as a surprise. Somehow though, holding the trifold paper in my palms and being able to touch the inked font with my fingertips, made it more real and shocking. The letter in my hands confirmed the inevitable I tried to escape daily.

My absences far exceeded the standard allowed by the school district and I was given only three options to choose from; return to school, become homeschooled by my parents, or become tutored at home.

I held my homework in my hands, bewildered, as I laid on my daybed—coated in brain fog and exhaustion. My backpack I once carried around school each day, I now could barely even drag across the floor. I looked at the all too familiar science lessons and math equations as if I had never in my life seen them before. I stared—for what seemed like hours— at the same page of my English book. I was unable to absorb the literature despite the dozens of times my eyes passed over the same sentences. My symptoms were so distracting.

I could barely see past the heavy stacks of papers that accumulated before me. I needed help if I was ever going to pass the seventh grade. It was clear in this moment that home tutoring was my only viable option.

Mrs. McDonald, my guidance counselor, was on the other end of the phone line as my mother explained to her that my mysterious illness was turning out to not be as temporary as we all hoped it was going to be. Mrs. McDonald was sad to hear that I would not be returning to school, but despite her disappointment, she supplied my mother and I with all the resources we needed to set up in-home tutoring. She served as a beam of light—one who guided us through the dim, confusing road towards my middle school education.

My pediatrician was required to fill out a form, explaining in detail why I could not physically attend school. The form was then dropped off at the school superintendent's office for review. Luckily—after anxiously waiting—my home tutoring request was approved by the superintendent and I was assigned a home tutor.

The day finally came—the day that my education would be resuscitated by my heroic tutor. I laid on my daybed in the dim-lit living room, encased in sheets and worries.

What if she's mean? What if she doesn't think I'm sick at all?

I asked myself many questions as my thoughts drifted back to my appointment with Dr. Stein, and all the past doctors who seemed to think I was the creator of my own illness. I began to grow angry with myself.

What if I'm really not sick, and I'm just creating all of this?

An aroma came from the neighboring kitchen and distracted me from my 'what if' thinking. I could hear the boiling water overflowing out of its pan and onto the stovetop as my mother juggled cooking dinner and cleaning the kitchen.

I was in the middle of a bad flare on this early evening in autumn. I felt overstimulated by the slightest of noises, even the faint sound of water boiling was too much to bear.

My mother's voice entered my fragile ears and jolted me from my daydream. My ear drums sputtered.

"C'mon Shay! I want you to get your schoolwork together so you're all ready for your tutor when she gets here!"

My intense detachment held me back, imprisoning me to my bed. My exhaustion held the key to my locked cell. I attempted to fight the hold, but I was still shackled by an intense pull of lightheadedness. It took great convincing for me to attempt to stand up, and even more for me to walk into the kitchen and sit upright in the wooden kitchen chair. Once I made it there, I closed my eyes and held on to my swaying face with my sweaty hands.

Why is sitting upright this uncomfortable and hard?

I struggled to grasp the reasoning behind it all. I felt like somebody was pushing me right out of my seat. It was becoming more and more difficult for me to sit upright at the kitchen table. Every minute that passed by seemed to bring with it a stronger pull from gravity. I swallowed the emotional lump in my throat, but it was climbing back up again. It was all just too much to take.

It was very dark outside as the clock pounded another hour. Headlights glared through the front porch windows, and my heart sank. My tutor was arriving, and in just a couple short minutes I would be meeting her. The doorbell echoed through the house as my mom walked over to the door and greeted my new tutor.

"Hello, I'm Mrs. K, nice to meet you," my tutor introduced herself.

An unfamiliar voice talked from behind the solid wood door.

"Nice to meet you. Come in!" my mother stated politely.

The two of them rounded the corner and into the kitchen. I was greeted by a tall, professionally dressed woman with medium length light brown hair. We spoke briefly about ourselves before Mrs. K reviewed the overwhelming piles of school work that suffocated our kitchen table.

She asked me many questions, but my body was becoming increasingly overwhelmed by my upright posture, making it very difficult for me to focus. My inclination to lay down was becoming more and more difficult to suppress. My eyes rolled harder and faster. The lump in my throat was no longer a tease. My eyes swelled in tears and I inexcusably walked swiftly back into the living room, without muttering a single word. I collapsed into the springy mattress of my daybed and hid my face as I sobbed in inconsolable grief.

At first my absence went unnoticed. I could hear my mother and Mrs. K talk about my schoolwork, as if I hadn't left at all. Soon though, they both rounded the corner into the living room and hovered over my ailing body. I could sense their stares and I could hear their conversation, but I was so overcome by symptoms that I could hardly engage. Mrs. K placed a gentle, concerned hand on my shoulder.

"I'm sorry you're going through this, honey. I hope you feel better," she muttered before leaving.

Her words touched my heart, even though I was too overtaken by symptoms to respond. I continued to cry and hide from my taunting realities. This was one of many evenings that produced unmanageable symptoms—I was always so much worse in the evening.

I didn't know it yet, but Mrs. K would pave the way for me for many years to come. This first meeting would not be the last. Mrs. K would be here for me for the long haul.

Chapter Five
Alone a Small Snowflake, Together a Snowbank

The walls of my chest feel like caving
Every breath is strong, but I can feel myself fading
Slowly, softly, and in the open
Vulnerable, tired, I'm so broken
I can barely convey my tragedy
I've lost myself, I've lost me
Can't you see that I cannot find
My health, my strength, my peace of mind?
I retrace my steps to see where I tripped,
But it appears I casually lost my grip

—"I Lost Myself" by Shayla Rose

I LAID SIDEWAYS in the recliner with my head and knees resting on each armrest. It was mid-morning in the early days of winter. I was so consumed. Devastatingly dying in plain sight. Tears filled my eyes. I didn't feel good, but after feeling this way for so long, I was sick of being sick. I was giving up more than I ever had before. My parents and Mrs. K stood beside me, asking me the same dreadful question as they had so many times before.

"What's wrong?" they asked.

I couldn't even respond.

What isn't wrong?

I had awoken on this winter morning in a fog of despair. I was floating through my life with not much more than a faint light to guide me. Or was it a light at all? I was unsure of so many things. I began to ponder my own self.

Who am I? Whose life am I living? Is living even worth it anymore?

I struggled to concentrate on my schoolwork, and as a result my tutoring session ended for the day. I was mad at myself for not focusing on my schoolwork—I felt like I had greatly disappointed those around me. But on this strange morning, I was consumed by strong emotions that I couldn't get a bearing on. I felt so ill, but I lacked the words to express my ailments. I felt so indescribably different. I felt lost, confused, sick, and scared.

A couple of days later, I sat in the recliner in my parents' bedroom, alone. It was the beginning of a snowstorm as I watched the snowflakes become illuminated in the beam casted by the outside light. The snowflakes drifted so effortlessly from the sky and gently blanketed the ground beneath. I was so mesmerized by each snowflake. I had seen snowflakes so many times in my life, but I had never paid such close attention to them before.

I was experiencing an awful episode of intense detachment—I could hardly distinguish reality from a dream. My hands didn't seem to be mine—my body was a stranger. I hadn't even eaten dinner, I was so dizzy that chewing food and struggling to swallow was entirely unappealing.

My mother soon came and sat beside me. Together we were wrapped in a warm blanket, watching the snowflakes reflect the light and fall carelessly to the ground beneath. Together, each snowflake made a difference, alone they were small and powerless.

We began to talk about the elephant that plagued our lives, about how my illness overcame me so suddenly and seemed to be in no rush to leave. We discussed my feelings of helplessness, and how not one doctor seemed to be willing to take me seriously. It was in this moment, surrounded by a blanket of warmth inside the depths of a chilling winter, I gave up.

"Mom," I said faintly.

"Yeah?" she responded.

"I can't live like this for another year, two years, three years—I can't live like this forever."

"I know baby."

"No!" I shouted, "I'm done!"

My mother took her hand and gently stroked my arm. In my mind my life was over, before it had even begun. I was just as alone as a single falling snowflake—powerless, small, and invisible. I didn't want to continue living, it was much too hard to continue facing my nameless illness.

"I just—I don't want to live anymore..." the words burned my mouth and left my throat stinging.

I was so sick, and help was so scarce. It didn't seem to matter how much water I drank, medication I swallowed or salt I sprinkled on my food—my life was unchanging in its demise. I was miserable, and I could not fathom the thought of facing years of the same intense symptoms. I wanted to escape it all—my detached body, my schoolwork, my ignorant doctors... my life. I was beginning to look at death as my only escape.

My mom held on to me and wrapped my broken soul in her love and warmth. We spent the next couple hours in this position as we watched the snowflakes outside coat the frozen ground. She knew I was giving up. For the first time in my life, my mom did not have the words to take the pain away. Instead, she just sat beside me and joined me on my roller coaster. She was unsure of it all too.

One afternoon, not too much later, my mother sat on the wooden stool in our kitchen with her laptop on the counter in front of her. She spoke a series of words I would not soon forget.

"Shayla! Come here! I think I found what you have."

I ignored her at first.

"Shayla, I'm serious! Come here!"

I got up slowly from my seat and hovered over her shoulder. I held on to the counter for support and sighed in defeat as she read me symptoms of some long-named, rare disorder I had never heard of before in my life.

"I doubt I have that!" I said to her before turning around and heading back to my seat.

On her laptop screen was a *Wikipedia* page titled "Postural Orthostatic Tachycardia Syndrome".

My mom continued to read information about this seemingly rare illness aloud, but I was only half-listening. In my broken mind, a diagnosis would never be found. As far as I was concerned, my mother was wasting her time.

What does Mom know? She's not a doctor. I'm so done—done with everything. Why should I believe what's written on the computer anyway?

My ailments painted a film over my view on the world. I couldn't see clearly anymore. My illness controlled so much of my life, I didn't even know who I was anymore. My hope was gone, but hers remained.

The days went on as my mother continued to present me with articles on this rare illness that plagued people all around the world. I didn't take her seriously—at least not until we were sitting on the couch together one day and the noise coming from her laptop caught my attention.

On the computer was a news story from Cincinnati. I was glued to my mother's laptop screen as I watched two young girls the same age as me mirroring my symptoms. They, too, had this long-winded diagnosis of Postural Orthostatic Tachycardia Syndrome.

My mother's face lit up. This, she was sure, was what I had. At first, I wasn't willing to accept that she was right. I had felt alone for too long, undiagnosed for too long, to believe that a name for it all even existed.

After a couple minutes went by, I was immersed in another video, this time of a nineteen-year-old girl who chronicled a day in her life as a POTS sufferer. It was while watching this video that I realized two things;

Mom might be right, and *I hope I'm not still sick when I'm nineteen.*

My mom made an appointment with my pediatrician and she presented my doctor with her research. But we left the office that day with frustration in our grip, my doctor had never heard of POTS before. She could not help me, and she made it sound like POTS was too far-fetched for me to possibly have. Even though I exhibited most of the symptoms of a POTS patient, my doctor left me feeling invalidated once more.

So... I have an illness that doesn't even exist?

I began to question everything, just as I had before. It was easier for me to not have any hope at all than it was for me to have my hopes crushed.

One night around dusk I sat on the linoleum floor in our kitchen. My tired back leaned against the cabinet doors. My heart raced, and I struggled to catch my breath. I felt increasingly detached from my surroundings and not one thing could bring me back. I was lost and drifting. The only words I could mutter other than,

"I don't feel good," was, "take me to the hospital."

I didn't like going to the hospital, but I was losing my grip. I was consumed by something greater than me, and nobody could tell me why.

After a long car ride, I laid on a white sheet on top of a hospital bed in the middle of the city. Tears slowly escaped from my eyes. I felt like I was balancing on a fine rope between consciousness and unconsciousness, and I was scared.
A nurse came and checked my vitals.

"Can you sit up for me?" the nurse asked.

"I feel like I'm going to pass out," I whimpered as I slowly sat on the edge of the bed with my eyes closed.

The nurse stood beside me as he placed a blood pressure cuff on my arm. He watched me closely, as though he was ready to catch my falling, lifeless body at any second. I never fainted, despite feeling so strongly that I would. My sustained consciousness seemed to puzzle my nurse, and he walked out minutes later with an annoyed gait. I almost wished in that moment that I had fainted, just to prove how sick I really was.

Soon, the doctor walked into the room. She greeted my parents and I and asked us some questions about my symptoms. After finding a doctor once again puzzled, my mother begged a question.

"What about POTS?" she asked.

The doctor gave my mother a confused gaze.

"Postural Orthostatic Tachycardia Syndrome?" my mother elaborated.

The best we could receive from the ER doctor that night was a 'maybe'. POTS was not ruled out, nor was it ruled in. We requested a heart monitor—as we had many times before—but our request was once again shot down. Because after all, my heart was fine, and I was 'healthy'.

I left the ER that night without a diagnosis.

"Stay hydrated and follow up with your pediatrician on Monday," the doctor instructed.

The car ride home was an emotional one. It was pitch black outside as I sat in the back seat of our Ford Taurus. My dad drove, and my mother sat in the back seat beside me. News headlines flashed in my mind.

"Local girl dies from mystery illness", "Girl goes to hospital and later dies, her family devastated."

I broke down. The fabric seats caught my tears. I was never this emotional—but I also never felt this misunderstood.

How can one of the best hospitals in the world shoo me out their doors without a diagnosis? How could they—people who save countless lives—be unable to save mine?

My thoughts were a jumble, and my emotions were weaved tight.

If it wasn't clear before, it was crystal clear now. We needed to find somebody who had heard of POTS if I was ever going to get better. Our search for a specialist would be time consuming, but my mother was not giving up. She was armed with as much motivation as a mother of a sick child could be and soon, she pulled out a doctor's name from the internet.

A day later, I sat on the grey couch in our living room, slowly pulling lint out of the arm rest. I rolled the tiny pieces of lint between my thumb and finger and squinted my eyes to get a closer look. Before long, my fit of boredom was no longer. My ears twitched, and I could hear half of the conversation as my parents went back and forth in the neighboring kitchen, discussing my health and the idea of taking me to a new doctor.

My mom picked up the phone and began hitting a sequence of buttons. Minutes later she came into the living room. She stood across from me with the phone still in her hand, a paper and pen in the other.

"You see the POTS specialist in May, okay?" she said with optimism.

My heart sunk, and I quickly shouted, "May?!"

Tears welled up my eyes and escaped over my lids. My cheeks were their runway as they gained speed before quenching the thirst of my denim jeans. May was four months away. I could never make it four more months.

How will I ever survive four more months without help? Will I really be left to fend for myself for four more months?

I laid on the couch crying as my gut filled with hopelessness. My parents attempted to reassure me.

"There's nothing else we can do but wait, Shayla. Hopefully this guy will really help you. Please don't cry!" my mother said.

My parents' comforting reassurance barely eased my broken heart.

Finally, after waiting for what seemed like forever, four months passed by and I sat down in a waiting room in the middle of the crowded city.

He spoke slow and dragged out. His voice was deep, and his analogies were confusing. The long-awaited doctor left me feeling guarded as he explained to me the anatomy of my illness and hesitantly confirmed our suspicions.

In a nut shell, I had POTS—although if you asked this cardiologist who sat across from me, he would likely string you along a confusing story about basketball players and you would forget entirely what your question was.

My blood was not returning to my upper body quick enough. Instead, it pooled in my lower extremities, causing debilitating dizziness as well as a host of other symptoms. The doctor wrote me a prescription for thigh height compression stockings and midodrine—a medication that works by narrowing blood vessels and raising blood pressure.

"People who take this medication tend to become bitchy," the doctor explained to my parents.

As a young lady with strong people-pleasing tendencies, 'bitchy' never fit into my vocabulary. 'Bitchy' was never an adjective I wanted my name to follow.

Although the doctor was sure that I had POTS, it was not the only illness he believed I was facing. He believed I also had Ehlers Danlos Syndrome, a connective tissue disorder that results in laxity throughout the body. Chronic Fatigue Syndrome was also on his radar, which explained my exhaustion. All these disorders were related somehow, they existed co-morbidly.

I tried the midodrine after much back and forth. I made it clear to my family that if I became snooty or rude, the medication should be stopped promptly.

I took one pill with flying colors. I felt somewhat relieved of my intense detachment, which was liberating to me, albeit short-lived. The side effects of the medication hit me early on. My head began to feel staticky, followed by intense, pounding pain. My body was overtaken by chills. I reached for a hat, I reached for a sweatshirt, I reached for pants in place of my shorts, then I needed a coat.

Before long I was standing outside on a ninety-degree day with mittens over my hands and layers of clothing covering my chilled body. I laughed at the sight of myself—I looked like a nesting hen in the middle of the Arctic, puffed up and ready to incubate anything that wished to sit still long enough.

The issue was not how I looked though. I didn't care if I had to buy out the entire winter section of the nearest department store, all I cared about was how I felt.

Off to the couch I went to sleep away my chills and pounding headache. Through the pain of my intense headache and through my double layered ski mask and scarf, I mumbled to my mom.

"I don't think I should take this med anymore."

It was with those words that we both realized it would be in my best interest to stop the midodrine. The compression stockings, however, would prove to be something I couldn't live without.

My mother took me to the closest medical supply store. We stood among walkers, canes, commodes, shower chairs, wheelchairs and other various medical devices as we waited for somebody to help us.

Eventually, a pleasant woman walked me and my mom to a small room in the back of the store and fitted me with compression stockings. I walked out of the store with black, thigh height compression stockings supporting my legs in a comfortable hug. They made my legs feel stronger and allowed me to stand for longer periods.

The box in my hands showed a picture of an elderly woman wearing her compression garments. Beside her sat her equally as elderly husband, both beaming with joy over the newest trend in compression wear.

Why, I wondered, *are most medical products geared towards the elderly? Not everybody is old who wears compression stockings!*

Chapter Six
Are You High?

Inside I am working, outside I am so still
Inside I'm on a roller coaster, except without the thrill
People watch me and wonder how I feel
Sometimes they just don't think my obstacles are real

— "Still" by Shayla Rose

ALTHOUGH I FELT LIKE I wasn't getting any better, over the course of several months, I was becoming less horizontal. A year after my initial onset, I was now relying less on my daybed, and was now able to stand and walk. It happened so slowly, and nobody could pinpoint exactly what had changed to promote my positive improvement. I found myself standing at the starting line of another school year—but this time, I was physically going to school.

My stomach was hard to hold. The swarm of nervous butterflies nearly carried me away. My legs shook in fear. I swallowed my cold water and sat in the passenger seat of our silver Ford Taurus bound for the junior high school.

Here I was, a year older and facing the same all too familiar brick building. I hesitated at first, my mind blocked my body from taking one more provoking step towards this educational dome, but with luring from my mother, I slowly began to move. The heavy metal doors swallowed me with one swinging gulp. I was inside now, and I was not allowed out.

I was not the same, happy-go-lucky, energetic teenager who once attended this school a short year ago. I looked at the world from a tainted lens. I talked with a sigh, and I avoided conversations at all cost. Eye contact was hard to hold, I felt unworthy of it. My illness took more than my health, it took my confidence too. This year would be different. Nobody knew me, I barely knew myself.

I was starting eighth grade with partial public school and supplemental in-home tutoring. Mrs. McDonald, my guidance counselor, helped me to receive all the accommodations I needed to get through my short school day without a hitch. In school I could have frequent snack breaks, water at all times, frequent bathroom breaks, and an elevator pass. My friend even kindly greeted me by the elevator every morning to ensure that my ride upstairs went as smoothly as possible.

"Welcome to eighth grade," my English teacher announced as I entered her brightly lit classroom on the second floor.

I glanced at her slowly, parted my lips into a half-grin and escorted myself to an empty desk. I placed my water bottle to my mouth before putting it on the top right corner of my wooden desk. I sat back in my seat, uncomfortable, and not familiar with a soul who surrounded me.

My ears filled with senseless chatter as my peers described their elaborate vacations and summer escapes. I spoke not a word. I simply sat and waited—all the while feeling increasingly isolated and awkward.

"Okay class!" my English teacher with blonde hair and plentiful excitement said as she closed the classroom door and walked to the head of the class.

In her hand she held a travel mug filled with her morning coffee. She introduced herself to the entire class and told us about her summer vacation before asking the class to do the same. Within minutes everyone got up and shifted seats. Everyone called to their friends and quickly sat beside them. It was in this moment that I realized, I knew nobody.

I felt like a grizzly bear who had entered hibernation, only to walk out of her den in the dawn of spring and realize she had slept through the entire next decade. Her surroundings changed, and she suddenly was the only animal in the forest she could trust.

I maneuvered slowly around the class before sitting beside a quiet girl. After a brief introduction, the girl asked me a hard to answer question.

"What did you do all summer?" she asked.

My mind drew a blank and before long I was smack dab in the middle of a long-winded explanation of my symptom provoking year.

"I feel like I'm in a dream all the time," I told her in part.

Her jaw dropped, and her eyes widened.

"That's terrible," she said sympathetically, "I couldn't even imagine that!"

I looked at her confused, my heart sank from her abrupt response. She looked at me with fear, as though the sensation of constant dreaming was the scariest thing in the world. My new normal had become a baseline of intense symptoms. I forgot in that moment, that feeling like I was dreaming all the time was not at all normal. The feeling of the world around me being a slow illusion was not a symptom that most people experienced, and my new classmate reminded me of that through her abrupt reaction.

Soon the teacher clapped her hands,

"Alright class, back to your seats!"

I was soon off to math class to witness a similar introduction and overview of the year. My math teacher was kind and to the point. She was honest—brutally honest—with a side of warmth we all adored.

My mind was heavy as I transitioned into the realm of eighth grade. I felt dazed, as if I was forever embraced by the cold shadow of my past. My body was fatigued, my limbs felt molded by concrete. My old life was gone—like a glass picture frame broken into a million ununiformed pieces, never again to be the same.

I struggled to speak to my peers, I couldn't relate to them. I was clamped in a trance of pity and self-doubt. I hated the world for continuing to thrive, because in my mind everyone else's world should have stopped when mine did. I spent the entirety of eighth grade in this morose state, unable to find the happiness I once wallowed in. I felt paralyzed amongst strangers, alone and defeated.

There was a conversation on one early morning in eighth grade that would stay with me for the next coming years. I walked into the small special education classroom and sat at a desk in the front of the room. Several classmates sat in the desks around mine, casually glancing at me as I made my entrance. I held my water bottle in my hand and a load of papers in the other. I could sense the stares of my peers and I slowly felt myself shut down. My sorrow-filled eyes stared at the tile, but my depressive stare was soon interrupted by a raspy voice coming from the desk beside mine.

"What's wrong with you?" a female voice asked before continuing, "Are you high?"

A lump entered my throat. My eyes widened. My heart skipped. I was taken off guard by this random voice. Nobody ever talked to me in school, and when they did, they never asked such blunt questions. I followed the voice and found myself looking into the eyes of a familiar red-haired girl.

"No," I replied, "I'm sorry, I'm just really dizzy."

I had never been asked if I was high before. My thoughts swarmed.

Do I really look like I'm drugged up?

The blunt red-haired girl and I ended up having a short conversation together, loud enough for the entire small classroom to hear. I explained my dreamy sensation to her and a brief overview of my medical past.

She looked at me with a puzzled grin and asked once more, "So does it feel like you're high?"

"I've never been high before," I claimed, "so I'm not sure."

The words from this red-haired girl echoed through my mind at the most unexpected of times in my life. I couldn't help but wonder how frequently she was high. She seemed to know the sensation too well to have not been.

Although this interaction left me feeling upset and shocked, it wouldn't be the only time in my life where I would be asked if I was on drugs. I suppose the fatigue that coated my

49

body, coupled with my slow response times and dazed expressions made some think that I was a drug user.

The autumns breath turned into a winter freeze, eventually replaced by spring flowers. Eighth grade had come and gone. Doctors had also come and gone. But my symptoms, although stable, remained.

Chapter Seven
Restoring Faith

I'm stronger than I thought, although my mind shatters
I have made it this far, and that is all that matters
My legs shake in weakness and dismay
But I carry the load one more day
My heart races right out of my chest
But I continue to carry on and do my best
The load may be heavy, your outlook grim
But your own light will guide you, no matter how dim

— *"Keep Moving Forward" by Shayla Rose*

I STOOD SHAKING as I maneuvered my way into the squeaky-clean high school. The floors were waxed, the walls were washed, and the entire school shined. A strong scent of cleanliness carried through the air, awaking the butterflies in my stomach. The school was prepared to welcome its annual round of naive freshman, and this year, I was one of them.

I spent the morning trailing around the high school with a handful of other students. We were led by a freshman English teacher—a man in his mid-forties—who briefed us on the basics of freshman year. I struggled to keep up with the pace of the group, and I struggled even more so to absorb the conversations going on around me.

I was so fatigued and overcome by symptoms that once we made it to the nearest classroom to look at the flashy new smart boards, I collapsed into the closest desk. The kids around me stood and looked at me as though I was being rude for sitting. I didn't care though. I drank some water and nodded my head slowly whenever the teacher looked at me. He talked about so many things, my brain simply could not keep up. It got to the point that I just stared at his energetic lips and completely tuned out his voice. Each time I thought the tour was finished, another student piped up with a question.

Soon, after what seemed like forever, the never-ending tour ended, and the entire incoming ninth grade gathered into the massive auditorium. The hallway leading to the auditorium was dim and narrow. My water bottle swung in my grip as I passed by several "No Food or Drink" signs.

I claimed a seat in a desolate location. Rows behind me sat dozens of rowdy boys, rows in front of me sat a group of unfamiliar girls. I was getting used to being alone, and I felt content by the emptiness of the surrounding auditorium seats. I became tangled in a mess of pitiful thoughts in this comfortable isolation, though, and I knew it wasn't healthy. I just couldn't relate to my peers, I was an outcast.

I watched an inspirational speaker prance his way around the high school stage on this late August day of freshman orientation. He encouraged the audience to get involved in his message and convinced us that we hold more potential than we may think. He proved to us that our minds are our biggest roadblocks and if we get out of our own way, we can accomplish things we once thought impossible.

I looked up at one point during this long speech to find an unexpected gesture. As if a beam of light shined at me through a foggy night, guiding me to refuge, a young girl stood rows ahead of me waving.

"Come here!" she whispered, her hand waving back and forth.

I shook my head no. I was hesitant to get up and greet her. I was not yet ready to move on and find new friends. I was afraid I would be rejected or misunderstood. My heart was simply too shattered to let anyone in. But, this girl two rows ahead of me was persistent. She continued to pry for my attention.

"Come here!" she pleaded once more.

My feet led my unsure mind as I slowly rose from my seat and walked to her.

"Hi Shayla!" she cheerfully greeted me, remembering me from kindergarten class nearly a decade ago.

"Hi," I responded hesitantly.

"This is my friend!" she said as she turned to the girl sitting on her left and introduced us to each other.

"Oh," I said awkwardly, "hello."

I was ready to retreat to the dark crevices of my existence. My eyes zoned in on my lonely seat two rows back and I became drawn to it like a magnet to a fridge.

"No, stay here with us!" my classmate insisted as she sensed my unsureness.

She patted the empty seat to her right. I sat down beside her and soon she handed me her cell phone number.
I left the presentation that day feeling as though I was rescued from the cold caves of my mind. I was given a kind dose of humanity when I needed it the most.

Freshman orientation wasn't over yet, though. My entire class quickly left their seats and spilled out of the auditorium doors like a swarm of bees leaving their hive. I slowly trailed behind. My nerves were bound tightly in my stomach, I felt so uncomfortable.

Lush fields laid in front of me. The warmth of the sunshine slowly melted away my nerves. I inhaled a fulfilling breath of cool morning air and felt my tense shoulder muscles relax. The open space of the outdoors was always calming to me.

A mixture of laughter and general conversation filled my ears in a steady murmur. Surrounding me were hundreds of my peers. Suddenly, one voice overcame the entire crowd and we all stood at attention, eager to receive the orders our teachers were about to present.

"Welcome to high school! Today we are going to be working on team building exercises! So, if you could all divide up in groups..."

My mind zoned out in worry as the teacher continued speaking.

Groups? Nobody is going to want me in their group!

I slowly wandered in to a crowd of unfamiliar faces and hesitantly engaged in awkward obstacles and team exercises until I drifted away from the kids completely. The energy levels of my peers were much higher than mine. I stood on the side of the field and watched from the sidelines, hoping that I wouldn't get in trouble for not fully participating.

I breathed a heavy sigh of relief when, off in the distance, I saw my mother pull in to the parking lot with her old silver Ford Taurus. I walked over to her and sat in the comfort of the passenger seat. It was finally time to go home. I could be myself in my mother's presence.

The mercury in the thermometer began to hold steady as I shut the screen door behind me and dismounted the three steps off our back porch. My parents sat outside under the shade of an umbrella in our backyard, and the phone sat on the metal table between them. Worry filled the face of my mother as the wrinkle between her brows became increasingly more prominent.

My mom had just got off the phone with the principal of the high school and learned that I would not be accommodated nearly as well as I was in junior high school.

"You can't be tutored and go to school," my mother said in part.

The high school relied on a new scheduling system, where every day was different, and each period rotated. It was called a block schedule, and this school year was the first time my school district was utilizing it. The unsteadiness that accompanied this new scheduling system made it virtually impossible for tutoring and partial school to be applied.

I was frustrated as I looked down at the brick patio in defeat.

"I can't go to school all day! That's—impossible!" I shouted to my parents.

But a week later I did just that.

My knees shook so violently they nearly gave me a black eye as I sat in the passenger seat of my mother's small car. The ride to school that morning seemed all too short and all too long. The closer we drove to the school the more violently my legs shook. Soon I could see the school in my sight, and the only thing between me and ninth grade was a line of puttering cars.

"I can't do this!" I whimpered to my mother in fear.

"You'll be okay," she reassured me.

I could tell my mother was almost as worried as I was.

The school was creeping closer, and soon I reluctantly got out of the car and walked inside. The hallways were filled with older peers I didn't recognize. As I walked through this unfamiliar scenery it was becoming increasingly obvious to me that I was lost. My stomach began to growl, and soon I was too cramped to even walk. I went inside of the nearest restroom, unable to make peace with my agitated stomach.

I was entering unchartered territory as I left the restroom and struggled to find the elevator. The white tile beneath my feet reflected the fluorescent lights from the ceiling, making every hallway look longer and narrower. The school bell chimed three times, and suddenly the crowded hallways were silent—the classrooms swallowed each soul within seconds.

I rode the elusive elevator up to the third floor and I walked even farther down vacant halls. I couldn't find my pre-algebra class—room 302—to save my life.

My heart raced as I imagined my new math teacher's disappointed face when I showed up to her class late. I felt like a fool, and finally, I gave up. I stood outside of an opened classroom door and sighed as I rounded the corner. I sighed so loudly that everybody in the classroom, the teacher included, stared at me with worry. It was in that moment that I read the sign outside the classroom door.

302

What a way to make an entrance. Embarrassed, exhausted, and with my pride left on the other side of the threshold, I took a seat.

At the head of my pre-algebra class stood my new teacher, Ms. Matthews, who was very young. Her age would prove to be her worst enemy as the students that surrounded me did all they could to overtake the classroom faster than a bad cold. She held her authority, though, despite my classmates' rowdy demeanor.

Hours later I was back at home, sitting beside my mother on the wooden bench in our vegetable garden, my first day of high school only a memory. She sat beside me with opened ears as I expressed to her the entirety of my first day.

I was accommodated well in the beginning of high school. I was able to eat my lunch in the quiet confines of the school therapy office—although in this setting I was mostly in the company of troubled teens, which made my lunch period socially uncomfortable. I wore an elevator key around my neck and was excused from physical education. I had two free periods every day, where I sat in Ms. Reed's resource room and made up tests and quizzes that I would inevitably miss due to the unpredictable nature of my chronic illness.

It was all going smoothly as I began to get used to the routine of full-time school. I was elated to be back in school where I belonged, but the friends I had when I was healthy were now complete strangers. I did not talk to them. My illness made me disappear for so long, that my friends' lives and routines began to function without me in them. I became replaced and forgotten.

Ashley—the friendly girl from freshman orientation—became my good friend. Somehow, our schedules were nearly the same, and because of this, we were able to spend a lot of time together. We maneuvered through freshman year by each other's sides. Without her, I'm not sure how I would have ever got through the day.

There was still something missing from my life, though. My classmates appeared to be wealthier than myself. Wealthy with friendships, social lives, independence, and health. I lacked the balance that they upheld. I could barely talk to anyone for the fear of what they would say in return. I lacked the ability to relate to my peers. I didn't find their jokes funny. I didn't find their behavior appealing.

I felt like I was the opposite of my classmates. I carried with me a heavy cloud of sadness. My past lingered over me and blocked out the light of every new day.

On one chilly morning in the middle of January, though, this all would change. The heavy storm cloud of my past would open up and melt my frozen soul with warm rays of light.

"Have a good day at school, I love you. Be careful on the ice!" my mother warned me before unlocking the car door.

A snowstorm had just passed days prior. Parking lots resembled skating rinks as the temperature plummeted below freezing.

I reached for the handle on the car door and I stepped out, preparing for yet another dreadful day of high school. But quicker than anticipated, my white sneakers slid on the ice. The world became a fuzzy blur and pain radiated from my butt to my head. I laid there, in the middle of the drop off circle in front of the high school, surrounded by dozens of onlookers. Embarrassment was an understatement as I felt the heat of my emotions warm my cold face.

Just as my vision began to clear, a hand appeared.

"Are you okay?" an older girl asked me as she grabbed my hand and pulled me to my feet.

"Uh...yeah," I said with a shaky stutter.

I grabbed my water bottle from beneath my mother's car, and the random girl handed me my snow-covered backpack before walking away. I followed her into the school with blood dripping from my palms. My head ached, my dizziness worsened, my heart pounded, but my soul warmed. Suddenly the heaviness of my past lifted. As I re-envisioned the unfamiliar hand lifting me from my fall, my faith in humanity became restored. It was in that moment—in the middle of the drop off circle at seven in the morning—that I realized compassion surrounded me. I was not as alone as I thought I was.

"Hi Ms. Matthews," I greeted my math teacher with tearful eyes, "can I use the bathroom to wash my hands?" I asked as I held out my scraped palms.

"Oh my!" she said with concern as she glanced at my bloody hands, "What happened?"

"I slid on the ice outside."

"Are you alright?"

"Yeah—I'm okay," I said through my shaky voice, "I just need to wash my hands."

I pushed on the swinging door and entered the brightly lit bathroom across the hall. I escorted myself to the sink, my body still trembling from adrenaline. I watched my blood swirl down the drain and the soapy water slowly lift away the dirt from my painful palms.

I glanced to the sink beside mine and spotted two familiar hands. I followed the hands up with my eyes and was led to a humble face.

"You're the girl who helped me!" I said hesitantly.

"Oh..." she responded slowly, unaware how far her kindness reached, "yeah! Are you okay?"

"Yeah, thanks for helping me like that," I said sincerely before leaving.

My tears of pain turned to tears of joy and warmth as I re-entered Ms. Matthews' classroom across the hall and sat in my assigned desk. As I found myself sitting in the middle of another bitterly cold New England winter, this unexpected, kind gesture would carry me through. It would carry me through like a lifesaver thrown to my drowning soul. Just in the nick of time.

Chapter Eight
Broken Trust

So tired, her energy taken
She was confused from the moment she'd awaken
She faces such struggle during the daily grind
She feels exhaustion from her feet to her mind
She is given two options between all that is left
She tries to decide which road leads her best
But one looks so rocky, the other so steep
Without much stability, which road should she keep?
She could continue down the road she is on
But the water is rising and soon the bridge will be gone
She cannot trust her skills to stay afloat
Not without the hint of a floaty, or the promise of a boat

— *"Exhausted Decisions" by Shayla Rose*

GOING TO HIGH SCHOOL full time every day became my default. I grew used to the long hours and tedious schoolwork. I was happy to be back in school, even though I often felt like an outcast beside my healthy and thriving peers. I felt pretty good, the best I had felt since becoming sick. I was proud that I was finally able to regain many of the abilities I had lost. This was all temporary, though, as I once again unexpectedly began to decline.

An awful cold struck me in early February, and while recovering, my grandmother took a fall. The stress that I underwent, both emotionally and physically was too much to take. Before I knew it, I was back at home, watching from the confines of my living room window as my neighbors got picked up by the school bus. I began to mumble words I thought I would never mumble again.

"I'm too dizzy to go to school," I told my mother.

The words that echoed through my hollow mind haunted me.

My mother's face drew worry as I now spent the better part of my days at home, hydrating and giving in to my body's fatigue. I had nothing else to do, but to give in.

Once again, my independence was yanked from beneath me. I felt like a beached boat waiting for high tide in the middle of a drought. Patiently I sat on the shore waiting. As the days went by my patience faded—the water simply would not rise.

Classmates would again stare at my empty desk with a distant memory of my quiet presence. Some may remember me on occasion, my existence being nothing more than a passing thought. Others would wonder who I was, unable to recall the name of the quiet girl they had never formally met.

After several weeks, a letter arrived in the mail, stamped with the public school's logo. I held my breath as I loosely gripped the trifold paper between my hands. I knew it couldn't be good—a letter from the school never was.

My absences from freshman year had accumulated and it was required of me to attend a meeting at the school. Except, of course, I was too sick to.

My mother attended the meeting at the school on my behalf several days later. Tutors slowly came back into my life as my mother negotiated with the high school guidance counselor.

Paula, my assigned counselor, agreed hesitantly to my mom's request for me to be tutored full time. It was simple, I was too ill to attend school. I had a doctor's note written by my pediatrician upon my request, and tutoring became my new normal. I was assigned three tutors during this time, who, for the next several weeks would help me continue my education.

One woman, Bettie, was elderly and had a pleasant demeanor. She had curly white hair and a contagious love for history and literature. My other tutor, Julie, was a young newlywed who was from the south and taught me physics. I also had another tutor, Anette, who taught me Spanish and algebra. She was very intelligent and guided me well.

The phone rang one afternoon, and Paula was on the other line. As my mother hung up the cordless phone, she shook her head in disgust.

"We have to meet with Paula next week," she began as she told me the details of the dreadful call, "and they want you to come in this time."

I was scared. My body was growing weaker as my illness began to slowly take control of me a little more each day. I was in no situation to prove myself to anyone.

After the week passed by, my mother and I reluctantly drove to the school. We walked into the therapy office where I once ate my lunch—the same small room where troubled teens vented to the school psychologist about their latest personal predicaments. The walls surrounding this room had undoubtedly heard a lot of heartbreak, and the carpet beneath me had caught many tears.

I sat at the head of an oblong table, although I might as well had sat on top. The discussion that was about to be had would leave me feeling like a turkey on Thanksgiving, unable to gauge where the next jab would come from.

My meeting was attended by the school psychologist Ms. Nicholson, my guidance counselor Paula, the assistant principal, my math teacher Ms. Matthews, and my extra help teacher Ms.

Reed, all of which had similar motives. Their job was to get me back to school, regardless of my physical condition.

"I thought I scared you with the letter I sent over February vacation!" the assistant principal jokingly suggested, "It seems like after I sent you that letter you didn't come back."

The assistant principal began to chuckle, but I didn't find his humor the least bit funny. I ignored him and turned my attention to Paula, who seemed to hold an ulterior motive behind her assertive posture.

"We want you to come back to school," she said in part, "you know tutoring is temporary."

Her point was clear. She did not want me to be tutored full time.

I looked around the oblong table into the eyes of my superiors, ashamed. Somehow, I had done something awful. Everyone seemed so disappointed in me. But what was it that I did?

I felt like a cigarette thrown out of a speeding car's window, left to smolder on the side of the road beside old scratch tickets and plastic bags. I was not worthy anymore.

The meeting ended with me following Ms. Reed downstairs to her classroom.

"So, here's your make up work..." she handed me a stack of papers and began to explain the details of each assignment.

I left with my pride tattered. Ms. Reed was changing, she was not the same lighthearted teacher I once knew and adored. Instead, she seemed upset. I wanted to please her—I wanted to please all my teachers—but I just couldn't.

After only a couple weeks of home tutoring, the high school's phone number showed up on our caller ID. Paula left a message on the answering machine, inviting me to a mandatory meeting with her and Ms. Nicholson. Although the intentions of this meeting were uncertain, I knew it wasn't going to be good.

"I bet they are going to make me stay!" I told my mom with tears threatening my speech.

I was sure that as soon as I entered the educational dome and was swallowed by the heavy metal doors of the high school, I would be forced to stay against my will.

"Don't worry about it," my mother attempted to reassure me.

When we walked into the high school on that early spring afternoon, my mother and I headed straight to the guidance office. It was a small room where seating was limited, and personal space bubbles were non-existent.

I battled so many emotions as I sat in that small room, surrounded by authoritative superiors. I felt guilty, as though my illness was a crime. I felt nervous, afraid of the unknown. But the one emotion that overcame them all was a nagging feeling of shame. I felt like a cowering canine with my tail tucked firmly between my legs.

Across from me sat Paula and to my right sat Ms. Nicholson. Their faces were that of sheer disappointment, and their voices grew sterner by the minute.

The air in the room was heavy enough to suffocate a human, the tension could have been cut with a knife.

I was so emotionally depleted. I struggled to comprehend their words, my concentration was non-existent as I tried desperately to fight through the fog.

"You need to come back to school," they said, "you can no longer be tutored unless you attend school."

Their words didn't make sense. If I could go to school full time, then tutors wouldn't be necessary. I tried to stand up for myself, but they would not listen.

By the end of the short, unbearably uncomfortable meeting, Ms. Nicholson escorted me to the resource room.

"I really don't feel well though, I—"

"You'll be fine," Paula said.

"I'm just so—"

"Come on Shayla," Ms. Nicholson stated.

I looked into my mother's eyes as long as I could, until she was too far away to see. My throat swelled with emotion, I could not speak. My lightheadedness grew as I walked down the long vacant hallways beside my authoritative escort. My stomach growled, although I couldn't decide if I was hungry for food or hungry for safety.

I rounded the corner into Ms. Reed's classroom. Rowdy students sat in chairs at the back of the room, studying for tests and playing on their cell phones. As I entered the classroom, they all stared at me intently.

I hid behind my long brown hair and sat quietly at a desk in the front row. I stared out the large window to my right. In my mind I envisioned my mother driving away in her car, leaving me behind in the confines of the high school.

I felt like I was jailed and forced to serve time inside of a prison cell. Every move I made became a written report. Ms. Nicholson quietly whispered to Ms. Reed before leaving.

My mind was so fogged, I could hardly fathom the thought of schoolwork. My small desk became full of papers as I completed tests and quizzes through my brick wall of impending syncope.

The school day was almost over, but one dreadful period remained. I wasn't comfortable knowing that as soon as the bell chimed, I would be expected to hike across the building to Spanish class. My legs felt so unsteady and my lightheadedness was unbearable. The long walk to Señor L's class seemed too far and unsafe for me to attempt.

I watched the second hand on the clock flirt with last period. I flinched as the awaited bell chimed. I packed up my belongings slowly, hoping that it would equal less time in my dreadfully overstimulating Spanish class.

"I don't think I can go to Spanish," I told Ms. Reed worriedly.

She was always so easygoing and understanding, but I was beginning to see a different side of her.

"You have to," she said with a seriousness I was not accustomed to.

My heart sank, and I bit my lip in hopes to get a better hold on my emotions. I wanted to cry so badly, but I couldn't show my weakness.

I paced myself as I walked to Señor L's Spanish class, battling the crowded hallways and waving occasionally to familiar peers. My heart was heavy as I walked through the door a couple minutes late. The kids around me did a double take. My desk had been unoccupied for so long that one kid began to use my chair as a place to drop his bag. Señor L gave me a familiar look of compassion and my worries faded briefly.

I completed my Spanish class and soon the school day was over. Relieved, I walked out of the confines of high school and into my mother's awaiting car.

Chapter Nine
Lighting up the Radar

Each day she wore her gloves, each day was a fight
She stared her illness in the face and stood with all her might
It was so difficult though, the challenges she faced
Inside of that ring, her troubles raced
She was punched with a dose of dizziness, and out of breath to boot
She was held by depersonalization, she could hear the crowds dispute
Her brain was foggy, she could barely even think
The referee banged the floor when exhaustion took the ring
She watched the crowds deplete, not many fans remained
She had very few friends, most forgot her name
Her illness was invisible to the naked eye
Most just couldn't understand why

— *"Boxing with an Illness" by Shayla Rose*

IT WAS JUST PAST seven o'clock in the morning as I navigated through the hallway on the second floor of the high school, trying desperately to be a normal student.

The fluorescent lights that casted life upon the long hallways seemed to become brighter and brighter. The steady murmur of the crowd radiated through my head and muffled out my own thoughts.

Suddenly, my vision blurred and the lockers that lined the hall were moving closer together, making my line of sight increasingly narrow. I became overwhelmed by my senses. Quickly I sat down on the side of the hall and closed my eyes. My weak body swayed, and my heart pounded intensely. I immersed inside myself as my body prepared to faint.

After a couple of minutes, I gained the courage to open my heavy eyelids. I looked around the blurry hallway and attempted to make eye contact with the moving crowd. I felt like I was lying at the bottom of a mob, and I hoped with all the faith in me that I would not get stepped on.

"Are you okay?" a voice said as an older girl made her way out of the crowd.

My heart became lighter as I found refuge in this kind student hovered over me.

"No, I'm really dizzy," I said with a great deal of distress in my voice, "could you walk with me to the nurse?"

"Yeah sure!" she said as she nodded her head and placed her belongings in a nearby classroom. "Here, let me take your bag," the girl offered as she lifted my heavy backpack and helped me stand up. "I'm Lily!" she introduced herself as we walked downstairs to the nurse's quarters.

I found out that Lily was the older sister of one of my classmates, and I thanked her profusely for being my morning hero.

"Hey Lily! Oh—hey Shayla," the school nurse, Mrs. Brooks spoke from behind her desk.

Mrs. Brooks voice faded to a pause as she stared at me. I walked by her desk and laid on the closest empty bed.

"She wasn't feeling well and—" Lily said before Mrs. Brooks cut her short.

"Yep, that's okay. Thanks for your help, Lily. You can go back to class now."

Lily shut the door behind her and headed back to class. Meanwhile, Mrs. Brooks turned her attention towards me.

"What brings you down here this morning Shayla?"

"I was walking down the hall and I got really dizzy. The hallways were so blurry, and I nearly passed out," I told her in part, still shaken from the close to unconscious excursion.

"Mmm... Hmm..."

A long pause lingered as Mrs. Brooks sat behind her desk in silence. I couldn't see her through the solid partition that separated us.

What is she thinking? She must not believe me. I'm going to get in trouble for coming down to her office so early.

My mind ran faster than a hamster on a wheel. My illness left me in a vulnerable situation. I could sense that trouble was brewing. Soon Mrs. Brooks broke the silence.

"It's so early!" she began, "School hasn't even started yet!"

"Yeah..." I said with a sigh.

What am I supposed to do? Wait until school starts? My illness doesn't know what time it is.

I struggled to get comfortable on the cold leather bed as I felt increasingly like falling to the floor. I felt like I was a marble on a ramp with gravity ready to claim me at any moment.

After a long, anxiety-filled wait, Mrs. Brooks emerged from her desk and walked around the partition. She spoke not a word as she sauntered across the room and grabbed the blood pressure cuff from the wall. She sat beside me on the leather bed and wrapped the cuff around my arm. Her stethoscope plugged her ears, and her eyes stared intently at the floor as she slowly began pumping the cuff with air.

The room was an uncertain silence.

"Your blood pressure is fine," she said, breaking the silence, "are you sure you are dizzy?"

I looked away, unsure of how to respond.

How can I prove to her I'm not faking it?

I truly felt like passing out, but my body showed no outward evidence.

"What do you feel like? I know you are dizzy, but what does dizzy feel like?"

She sat on my bed and begged for answers. Answers I did not hold.

I felt like my symptoms were being doubted. Mrs. Brooks knew I had POTS, but this loose diagnosis was not enough. POTS was nothing more than a random abbreviation. It was too "rare"— something I couldn't possibly have, at least not without plummeting blood pressure.

"Um..." I began, "ah..."

I couldn't find the words. Adjectives left me stranded mid-sentence and I felt like a stuttering fool. My chest tightened as the pressure of her stares interrogated me.

She continued prying for answers until finally I dropped a word that would change my entire high school world forever.

"I feel like I'm in a dream. It's called depersonalization."

I released the word like a bomb. Quickly I watched the shrapnel from the word wound my authenticity.

"Oh! Well why didn't you just say that!"

With that one sentence Mrs. Brooks jumped up from my bedside and walked back to her desk.

I could tell from her face that she received just the answers she was looking for. This sentence confirmed to Mrs. Brooks that my illness was more psychological than physical—that I was simply so anxious that I made myself physically sick. The keys on her keyboard began to click something fierce. I knew that I was in trouble.

I unzipped my backpack and began to drink my juice box. I placed pretzels in my mouth, hoping that the salt would save me from the brink of unconsciousness.

I untucked my cell phone from the front pocket of my bag and I secretly texted my mom. The solid partition that stood between me and the desk of the nurse now served as a comforting armor against her blank stares.

I'm very dizzy. In the nurse. Will u pick me up?

My mom responded quickly.

Ok be there in a minute.

I felt so disconnected from myself and from the world around me. My whole body was fatigued, and I felt so lightheaded.

Mrs. Brooks stood up from her desk and walked to the end of my bed.

"Okay Shayla! Ready to go back to class?"

"I'm too dizzy," I claimed.

"No, you'll be okay," she attempted to reassure me as the bell chimed for second period.

"My mom is on her way to pick me up. I'm going home," I told her.

"Huh?"

"I texted her." I held my maroon LG phone in my hand, and a small smirk overcame my face.

Mrs. Brooks expression changed quickly. She walked away from me and retreated to her desk. The tense silence in the room now grew even tenser as I quietly waited for my mom to arrive.

"Shayla your mom is here," Mrs. Brooks mumbled.

"Okay."

My mother met me in the main office and together we left.

The days went by slowly for me as the mood in the nurse's office days prior sat in my mind like a bad house guest that wouldn't leave. I became frustrated with myself for speaking too much, but there was nothing I could do. The word was already dropped, the damage was already done.

Inevitably so, I ended up back in the nurse's office just days later. This time though—just as suspected from her body language during our last encounter—Mrs. Brooks wasn't happy.

I sat in Ms. Reed's classroom, unable to concentrate on my work. The more I allowed my eyes to scan over pages in my textbook the more intense my symptoms became. I could hardly comprehend where I was through the thick detachment that coated me. I didn't feel safe—I felt like passing out and I was in no setting for it.

I pumped my ankles up and down and I massaged my aching thighs. I tapped my feet against the tile floor, and soon I just couldn't take it anymore.

I stood from my desk and walked to Ms. Reed who was at hers. She looked up at me with distrust in her eyes, as if she knew my words before I did.

"What's up?" she asked, looking disinterested in our conversation as she gazed around the classroom.

"I really don't feel well. Could I please go to the nurse?" I begged.

She bit her lip, "Are you sure?" she asked, as if my symptoms were open for negotiation.

I nodded my head yes.

"Okay then," she said hesitantly while she scribbled a note and placed it in my palm.

I turned around and grabbed my backpack. The heat of my emotions made my forehead overheat. I glanced at Ms. Reed— who was now on the phone—and I shook my head. Her phone conversation was too quiet for me to hear. I didn't have to hear her though, I already knew what she was up to.

I walked into the hall with my head draped down in shame. I never felt more alone. I felt my confidence and self-worth unravel as I rounded the corner into the nurse's office once more. I felt like I was a criminal.

Mrs. Brooks was on the phone as I entered the room. I had a good idea who she was talking to, and her tense stares confirmed my assumptions.

I found myself a bed on this mid-morning in spring and I dropped my heavy backpack to the floor. I could feel a shaky unsureness overcome my body. I was so alienated and alone here—inside of this high school that so many townsfolk praised.

As my thoughts drifted downward into a spiral of worry, a loud click brought me back to reality. Mrs. Brooks hung up her phone forcefully.

A couple seconds of awkward silence ensued before the solid partition began to speak.

"Feeling dizzy again Shayla?" Mrs. Brooks said, reaping sarcasm and in no rush to come check on me.

She stayed at her desk, clicking away at her computer, seemingly awaiting the arrival of somebody more important.

"Yep..." I said with unsureness.

Moments later, after many of my fingernails littered the floor, Paula came in.

"Who's here this morning?" she asked, as if she didn't know.

"Shayla," Mrs. Brooks responded, "you know Shayla."

Paula's presence in the nurse's office was unusual. This rare appearance from my guidance counselor was a red flag. I knew I was in trouble from the moment I heard her voice.

"So, you're feeling nervous?" Paula asked me, intimidating me with what seemed to be a staring contest of eye contact.

"No, I'm dizzy!" I responded.

"It's okay to be nervous."

"I'm dizzy," I said again.

I began to feel like an unarmed horseman in the middle of a jousting match. The jabs of Paula's lance were coming at me, but I had no lance to fight back with.

"Well I looked up depersonalization. You need to stop reading about it online," Paula told me as she looked directly into my eyes.

My heart sank.

"It's not like that!" I told her, as I began to get angered.

I didn't know what to say, my mind went blank as it thrashed in emotions. Nothing that I could say would change her mind. But her opinion didn't matter to me, it was her authority that scared me.

I suddenly felt so betrayed by Mrs. Brooks. I had a physical medical condition, and—although debilitating in its own right—I was not suffering from a bad case of anxiety like Paula persistently implied. I began to feel so uncomfortable as I realized how much of my medical information Mrs. Brooks shared with Paula. I trusted Mrs. Brooks with my symptoms, and she broke my trust and used my symptoms against me.

Paula began to go back and forth in conversation with Mrs. Brooks at my expense. Their voices were loud as they talked about my symptoms. They went on and on, as though I misled them and disowned them the entire year—all because I was depersonalized. They made me feel like a fraud.

I texted my mother—somehow—during their fury. I hoped with all my faith that my mother would once again be my last-minute safety net and save me from any more jabs from Paula's lance. I honestly had no other options, I needed to escape. I didn't feel safe.

I'm here, my mother texted me as she sat in the main office of the high school.

I got up and packed my bag and walked right past Mrs. Brooks desk.

"Where are you going?" she asked.

"I texted my mom and she is here to pick me up," I said, my chest bound so tightly with emotion I could barely speak.

I walked away without looking for further approval. Her opinion didn't matter to me. I knew from my history, from my doctors' notes, and from my symptoms that I was sick. I needed support and encouragement as a teenager with chronic illness, but instead they gave me sarcasm and invalidation.

I walked to my mom as she stood calmly in the main office. Seeing her face was like seeing a long-awaited beam of light after a very dark night. Finally, I felt safe. She looked into my eyes and could see the obvious distress I was under.

"Are you okay?" she asked me before walking out of the main office.

I could not speak, I was much too shaken. I led her out the heavy doors of the high school and walked to the car. My body was so tense, and my adrenaline surged.

"What's wrong?" she asked me once more.

"I don't know!" I responded as my voice weakened and my head shook in disappointment.

As soon as I sat inside of my mother's car, tears ran from my eyes like a rushing river. I moaned inaudible words through my meltdown of disbelief. I struggled to piece together what had just unfolded in the last hour. My emotions weighed on my mind so heavy that my brain was now exhausted. My mother was confused, as she only caught bits and pieces of my emotional meltdown.

Not too much later that day, my tutor Anette came to my house to teach me algebra and Spanish. I sat beside her, tight lipped. I answered her questions about my school work with short, one-word responses. I was so depleted and closed-off—a far cry from my usual outgoing self.

Soon, Anette caught on to my odd behavior and asked sincerely about my well-being.

"Bad day at school?" she asked.

I nodded my head violently before collapsing it into my palms. Anette's one question broke my composure like a needle to a water balloon. The emotional waves of tears just kept flowing and I could not stop them.

My mom came into the kitchen, concerned about what she overheard. She quickly came to my side.

"What's wrong?" my mom asked me, placing her hand on my shoulder.

But I could not respond. I felt far too betrayed, far too overwhelmed, to even form a word. My hands were drenched in tears as I hid my face behind them.

"I think I opened a can of worms," Anette said to my mother, "I asked her how her day was."

"Yeah. They have been giving her a hard time," my mother stated, referring to the school system.

My tutoring session stopped short as I struggled to gain my composure. I hurried into the living room and laid face down on the couch. I shouted out every detail of my day to my mother who sat beside me.

"I feel like I'm on the radar. I'm not going back there! Please don't make me go back!"

My rant continued through my tears as my mother gently rubbed my back.

"You don't have to go back," my mother said, showing displeasure over the way the school treated me. Our conversation continued in great length.

I never would see Anette again. In fact, I never would see any of my tutors again.

Chapter Ten
Picking up the Pieces

I sat in an empty room, quiet as could be
With my future a pencil stroke away from me

— *"Relieving the Pressure" by Shayla Rose*

THE PHONE RANG after I didn't show for school. I didn't even want to know what the school had to say. No matter what I did I would never be able to change Paula or Mrs. Brooks mind about my illness.

My chest ached, and my heart hurt sharply. I was so mentally overworked that I thought my mind was going to explode. The stress that the school officials casted on me was too great to handle, and it was only about to get worse.

Paula called and stated that the school would now revoke my tutors due to me not returning to school. With five weeks remaining in my freshman year, my in-home tutoring was terminated. My education—pulled from beneath me.

The same local high school that received immense praise for its graduation statistics, did not care how I would receive my diploma.

I had so much anger flowing through my veins after hearing the details of the latest phone call from Paula. I went through the motions of living every day, but I didn't feel alive. Stress consumed my every cell. My mind was so consumed with thoughts of worthlessness. I felt guilty. Even though my illness was very real, I couldn't help but wonder if it was all in my head like so many suggested.

"Now what?" I said to my mother as I sat on the recliner in her bedroom, the chair rocking violently with each push of my foot to the carpeted floor.

"Well you'll have to be homeschooled I guess, Shayla. I don't know," my mother stated, furious that I was denied my education.

My mom was just as overwhelmed as I was.

"I'm going to have to return these," my mother said, days later while holding my textbooks in her hands.

Paula made it clear through the latest phone call that all my textbooks had to be brought back to the high school promptly. Not only were my tutors taken away, but my books soon would be too.

We began a desperate search to find the most effective way for me to be homeschooled. I was underage—only fifteen at the time—so quitting school was not legal nor something I wished to do. I wanted to be able to graduate. My illness had already taken so much away from me, I wasn't about to let it take my education away too.

I sat in front of my mom's laptop for hours with my mom, desperately searching for curriculum. We hardly knew where to begin, having neither of us played the role of teacher before. Eventually, we found a couple of websites and printed off pages of high school appropriate worksheets and quizzes. *YouTube* became my teacher. My empty living room became my classroom.

After several weeks of homeschooling in my quiet living room, I finished freshman year and found myself in the early days of summer break. The haunting question remained though, how would I graduate?

"How will I graduate?" I asked my mother as I stared out the open window in her car, the wind hitting me in the face.

"You'll have to get your GED," she answered.

"No! I don't want that!" I shouted as I became angered in defeat.

Nothing was going right. I was an exhausted, sick teenager with no social life. I felt accused by doctors and school officials of causing my own illness and now—as if all of that was not enough—I had to settle for an equivalency diploma? The entire world seemed to stand against me.

Getting a GED was always frowned upon throughout school. This argument between my mother and I quickly took me back to a couple of months prior, when I sat in the quiet library of the high school. I was working on a school project at the time, when I overheard a conversation between an older student and her guidance counselor.

"Kaitlyn! You have to do your work. Come over here!" the counselor told her in a voice too loud for library standards.

"I'm not going to stay in school anyway. I'm just going to get my GED!" the girl shouted in anger, unwilling to bow her head to the cookie-cutter lifestyle that the high school handbook seemed to project.

"That won't get you anywhere!"

The girl eventually walked over to the counselor and reluctantly completed her schoolwork.

After overhearing this conversation, it took a lot of persuading for me to understand that earning a GED was not a shameful thing.

All summer from my air-conditioned house, I studied for my General Equivalency Diploma. I read the large GED study book from cover to cover, took notes and carefully completed every worksheet.

Finally, in the early days of fall—weeks after my sixteenth birthday—I took the test.

"Well, we are here," I said to my parents from the back seat of the car, my legs trembling in fear.

"You'll do good, kid," my dad reassured me.

We drove nearly an hour to a certified high school that offered GED testing. A large banner flew in the breeze, "#1 High School of 2013". I looked at the banner with a comforting smile as I began to scan my surroundings.

In front of the school ran dozens of pupils following closely together in a unified group. Some students smiled and joked while most others took the after-school track practice much more seriously.

I gripped my trusty stainless-steel water bottle in my hand—the same one with large dents in it from my faith boosting fall on the ice—and I walked alongside my parents to the entrance of the well honored high school before me.

The security guard was expecting us. He asked for my ID and unlocked the front doors to the impressively large school.

I stood in the broad lobby as I talked to my dad nervously. My voice carried through the lobby with a clear echo. The security guard escorted us down short brick hallways and soon brought us to a small office with two desks and a round table in the center.

"Hello, I'm here to test for my GED," I said hesitantly.

Two women sat at separate desks in front of me, both with intimidating, frozen expressions I only hoped to melt away.

"You must be Shayla," one of the women said, her dark hair curled to just above shoulder length, "The instructors will come and get you shortly, you can have a seat."

My parents and I sat together at the small round table in the center of the room. I unzipped my bag and began to drink my orange juice, in hopes that the sugar would give my fading body an extra boost of energy.

My father made general conversation with the two receptionists as, he too, attempted to break their iced expressions. My dad always started small talk with strangers. Usually his method began with general topics like the weather, or by making observations in the room.

"That's a wicked cool stapler, I've never seen one like that before!" he began.

I sighed nervously to my mother and looked into her eyes.

"You'll do fine," she reassured me as she squeezed my cold hand.

The wait seemed like forever on this fall evening in 2013. I felt as though in these paused moments, I was holding both my past and my future at the very same time.

Footsteps and a squeaky door suddenly broke my deep thoughts. I glanced up and greeted my two professors.

"Hello, I'm Henry!" an older gentleman with a balding head shook my hand before turning to my parents to shake theirs.

"Hello, I'm Judy, nice to meet you all!" a tall, middle-aged woman introduced herself.

After a brief overview of what to expect, Henry and Judy led me to a private classroom. The process of getting my GED was a lengthy one. Every subject had separate tests and each test took a long amount of time to complete. The entire test was six hours long. Luckily, I was accommodated well and able to divide up my test into three sessions.

By the end of each test day, I was too dizzy to walk a straight line and too fatigued to hold a conversation.

We traveled back to this well-awarded high school on three separate occasions before the silent wait for results began.

The weeks passed by slowly, until one day when my mother shouted at me through the back door of our house.

"Shayla! Hurry up!" my mother yelled as I stood outside in the backyard, attempting to busy my under-stimulated mind.

I rushed into the house as fast as I could, fearing the worst. Her tone sent chills down my spine. My mom rarely yelled.

"You got your GED!" she excitedly shouted as I opened the back door and stood in the kitchen.

I jumped and twirled as my voice grew weak with emotion and tears filled my eyes. As the words left my mother's lips, I felt the heavy weight I had been carrying since my high school days lift. Finally, the dark days of high school could be buried by my successes.

My mom replayed the message on the answering machine of Henry—my instructor—telling me my results. Soon my dad came home from work and we told him the good news, too.

"No way!" my dad said as he took his coat off and laid it on the kitchen chair.

He asked me for a high-five and praised me for my hard work.

It was an interesting phenomenon, to be a sixteen-year-old with a diploma. In many ways I was now ahead of my peers, although my illness still made me feel behind.

Darren,   Apr 29, 2019

I hope you enjoy reading my book. I wrote it to help spread awareness about POTS and to help others feel less alone. If you enjoy the book, please leave a review online at www.blazingtrailspublishing.com or on my goodreads or FB page.

Thank you. I hope you are doing well!

Love,

Shayla ♥

Chapter Eleven
Now What?

The large wooden door slowly crept shut
She could sense it in her soul and feel it in her gut
The latch clicked, but she had not a single key
She lifted her fist to knock but stopped herself mid-plea
As the light of her past faded to dark
She sat alone, in darkness, longing for a spark
Just then, she heard a subtle crack
She shivered as a breeze tickled up her back
A window opened slowly, the curtains blew
She started towards it and then right through

— *"When God Closes a Door, He Opens a Window"* by Shayla Rose

I STARED AT my diploma on the kitchen table. My smile had an unsureness behind it. I was happy to have earned this one-way ticket out of high school, but I was equally as concerned. All my studying had led to this moment, sitting in my quiet kitchen as a graduate.

I felt just as alone in my success as I had in my darkest times. My parents praised me, my grandmother cheered. My family placed a cake in front of me and I received a nice card and a cute figurine, yet I sat there with a great deal of uncertainty. I had now permanently removed myself from the setting of school—removed forever from the engagements of my classmates.

What do I do now?

I sat in my living room, alone with myself and my future. I took a sip of water out of my old, dented brown thermos and I focused my attention on my laptop monitor. Ever so carefully I scrolled down pages of job postings, waiting for one to catch my eye. My job search became a job.

I couldn't wait to start working, I was so eager to get a fresh start outside of school. What I didn't know, was that the workforce was remarkably similar to school. Having a chronic illness was not always going to be well understood, or well accommodated.

Several months after getting my GED, I got hired to work as an assistant at a local childcare program. I enjoyed my time there, but after a couple months, I decided the job was no longer for me.

A couple of months later I got hired to work inside of a warehouse picking orders. I could only work a couple of hours per shift before my symptoms became too intense, but luckily short shifts were just what my employer was looking for.

Although my shifts were short, my body just barely managed to get through. Every day I would come home in an exhausted fog. After a quick snack I would stumble to the couch and drift off to sleep, but no matter how much I slept I did not feel rejuvenated. My entire day after a shift was ruined as my body attempted to regain its strength and replenish its depleted energy reserves.

I never missed a day of work despite my illness. I walked all around the warehouse with my skipping heart. I swept my fatigue and depersonalization around with every stroke of the broom against the warehouse floor. My blood pressure dropped with every pick of an order.

I knew that if I was ever going to last working anywhere, I needed to heed the warnings of my body. When my body demanded water, I gave it some. When my body began to overheat, I took off my sweatshirt. When my heart rate got too high, I slowed down my pace.

Sadly enough, these self-made accommodations became an issue and I learned firsthand what work place discrimination looked like.

"Go and dust off those shelves and products for me," my manager gave me clear orders, as she handed me a duster.

I stood on a step stool and worked at my own pace, thoroughly cleaning off every dust bunny and dirt particle that my naked eye could see.

I worked diligently for what seemed like a half an hour before I became completely overtaken by my symptoms. Lightheadedness tried to throw me off my step stool with every chance it got. Working with my arms above my head made my heart pump faster and harder, making me feel increasingly like passing out. I tried to ignore my symptoms at first, but soon I had no choice. I looked down at the concrete floor beneath me and I shook my head.

It isn't worth falling, Shayla.

I needed to accommodate the situation if I was ever going to get my job done in a safe and timely manner.

I took all the products off the high shelves and I lined them on top of a cart in front of me. I used my step stool as a seat and I sat there dusting products, alone with my thoughts as I adapted my task to become more POTS friendly.

Just as I was getting into a steady groove of dusting and cleaning, a loud conversation broke my focus. The warehouse manager walked past me with her cell phone pressed firmly against her ear.

It was clear that my manager was speaking to someone important as she offered very few jokes and talked strictly business. Her hands waved in all directions as she paced the concrete floor.

Just as she walked away, and her voice grew fainter, my ears twitched once more. She was turning around and heading back in my direction.

"No! Don't do that!" she shouted at me exhaustedly through her important phone conversation, "Yeah, yeah. Right, well those orders are..." her voice grew softer as she returned her focus to the person on the phone and walked away.

I looked at my step stool that was beneath me, the clean products in front of me, and the shiny shelf above me. Then I looked back at my manager. I could not understand what I was doing wrong, so I continued working.

Minutes later my manager hung up her cell phone and started a seemingly endless rant.

"You cannot sit on the job! Okay? It doesn't look good. If somebody walked in here right now, they would think you were being lazy and didn't care. Got it? Here, let me see this," she reached out her hand and grabbed the duster before changing her tone, "When you sit here like this, it says to me that 'I am lazy, and I do not care about my job. I am just sitting here dusting away because there is nothing better for me to do, and I do not care.' Whereas if you stand while dusting you look like you are working. Got it?"

She handed me back my duster and stared at me as I failed to fully express how I felt.

The emotions within me were heating me up like a compost pile. I wanted to scream, I wanted to cry, but instead I

94

did nothing. It was easier for me to just agree with my managers opinion than it was to fight it. So, I sat there and heard her out while biting my lip and attempting to calm my aching heart.

I was tired of being shamed for things I didn't do wrong. Instead of observing the great job I did dusting the shelves and products, my manager instead chose to focus on the fact that I was sitting while doing it.

I was more than once misunderstood by this warehouse manager, who seemed to believe that illness and laziness were interchangeable words. I quit my job days later.

This warehouse position would not be the last time I encountered work place discrimination, though. Months later, I applied for another job at a new business just a couple of towns away.

I sat across from a middle-aged man and woman as they interviewed me and my mom for their newly posted job positions. They operated their business at an old warehouse, and the job entailed cutting and packaging food.

We discussed the job in detail, and —at the risk of ruining the entire interview and any chance of getting the job—I told my potential future employers about my illness. I wanted to be upfront with them.

"I have an illness called POTS. I'm not sure if you've heard of it before, but basically my blood pressure gets low and I have to sit down frequently. It can be hard for me to stand for long periods because of my dizziness. I'm a hard worker though, and my illness isn't as bad as it used to be."

The employers looked at each other and then turned back to me.

"That shouldn't be a problem, we have a couch in the break room. Anytime you have to lie down or take a break, go for it."

My mom and I left the job interview with a handshake to our hosts, and shortly thereafter our phone rang. We got the job.

Day after day, I used a knife to cut food and package them up for grocery stores. Each shift was four hours long, with one fifteen-minute break in between. I worked so hard there. I pushed myself hard to ensure that my illness didn't affect me from completing my job duties. But it all ended in an instant, on one average afternoon.

I was finishing packaging up a food order when my boss asked me for help.

"Hey Shayla, when you're done with that would you mind helping out Emma?"

"Sure," I responded.

I walked over to Emma who spoke very little English. She stood across from me at a table as we both quietly cut and packaged a large order. I stood and helped her well into my break, but soon my symptoms overtook me like a heavy wave. I tried to ignore my symptoms at first, but the floor was coming closer by the second and my legs grew more and more unsteady. I looked up at the clock and then I looked back down at the table in front of me. My body needed hydration and food. It was already nearly an hour past my scheduled break, and I was going to pass out if I continued. As much as I wanted to ignore my symptoms, I couldn't. I had to say something.

"I didn't get to take my break yet. I'm really dizzy, is it okay if I go take one and then come back and help you?"

"Yes!" Emma said with enthusiasm and an eager nod of her head.

After telling my supervisor and getting her permission, I clocked out at the time clock. As I turned around to head to the break room though, my boss blocked my way.

"Where are you going?" she asked angrily.

"To take my break. I didn't get to take it at two o'clock," I told her as I struggled to suppress my intense symptoms.

She shook her head no. It was clear she wasn't happy.

"You really can't do that if you are helping somebody," she said.

"Well, if I don't take one, I'm going to pass out," I walked past my boss, without looking for her approval.

It didn't matter to me what anyone said. My symptoms were not up for debate. It was simple, I needed to take a few minutes to eat something before somebody was picking me up off the floor.

During my break my boss watched me closely. She paced in and out of the break room, as though there was something she wanted to tell me. She never spoke though, instead she just watched me intently.

Once my break was over, I walked back to the time clock and my boss pulled my mother aside.

"I really don't think she should work here. Especially if she gets dizzy," she told my mom.

It was in that moment that I was again discriminated against. Despite my employer knowing about my illness well before hire, she chose to fire me for it.

I took a break from working for a couple of months as I needed to emotionally and physically recover from my experiences. It was during this recovery though, that I encountered a new health issue.

Chapter Twelve
Expect the Unexpected

Wrapped in a gown
Silently I plummet down
The ones around me do not see
That something great is taking me

— "Fading Out" by Shayla Rose

"HEY THERE, I'M LEANN one of the providers here," a middle-aged woman with medium length brown hair and a white lab coat introduced herself. "What's been going on?" she asked.

"Well my left side hurts. I'm pretty sure I have an ovarian cyst," I began, "I need to have an ultrasound."

Leann seemed leery of my sureness, clearly it wasn't every day that somebody came into the clinic telling the doctor what tests to order.

We went back and forth in an educated discussion. Leann believed I was perhaps constipated, which—given my history of Irritable Bowel Syndrome—was not a far-fetched diagnosis.

I held true to my instincts though, and I continued to ask for an ultrasound. I had experienced ovarian cysts before, so I knew what they felt like.

"I really think I have a cyst," I told Leann.

Leann bit the inside of her cheek and looked at me for a couple of seconds.

"Okay, I'll go order the ultrasound. I'll be right back," she said.

Leann returned, my ultrasound was scheduled in an hour and I had to fill my bladder up quick.

After drinking myself to the verge of peeing, I walked next door for my appointment at the radiology suite. The technician performed my ultrasound and sent me back to Leann so she could read me the results.

Leann walked into the exam room with a smirk. I laughed at her expression, I knew what she was about to say.

"Well you were right," she said with laughter, "you have a cyst on your left ovary."

She went into details on the size and type of my cyst before sending me and my mother home.

"Have some ibuprofen for discomfort, come back if it gets worse," she said to me as I grabbed my bag and began walking out.

"Okay thank you!" I responded.

Typically, ovarian cysts disappear on their own—many women don't even realize when they have one. My cyst was stubborn though, and it just kept growing.

Each day I was in more pain. My left side, right near my hip, felt like the combination of a strained muscle, and a bad cramp. It continued to get more debilitating as time progressed, and before long I found myself at the local hospital.

I was so nauseated as I sat in the middle of the cold ER waiting room around midnight, my parents on either side of me.

We waited for what seemed like an eternity before I couldn't wait any longer.

"I have to use the bathroom!" I told my parents in an urgent tone.

I walked to the ladies' room and then returned to the waiting area where a miserable triage nurse greeted me.

"You aren't supposed to use the bathroom, eat or drink anything if you are in the ER for abdominal pain," she told me sternly before checking my vitals.

I'm not sure what this triage nurse expected of me, but when nature calls, nature calls.

I was sent back into the cold ER waiting room where I watched the clock tick by. It was now three in the morning and nobody was calling me in.

Many doctors went home for the night and—due to the large volume of patients and small volume of doctors—many patients spent the night in hallways instead of rooms, where they would wait for several more hours until the morning shift arrived to tend to their emergency needs.

We ultimately went home without seeing a doctor, finding it to be wiser to sleep at home than in a cold hospital hallway.

I soon decided I would just live with my intense discomfort. Having sought help at the local hospital just days before and being pushed aside, I figured I could cope okay at home.

I was tired of the pain, but I was equally as tired of the lack of treatment I was receiving. I wasn't sure at that point what was worse—having a growing cyst overtake my ovary or going to a hospital where I would ultimately feel shamed, misunderstood, and invalidated.

My stubbornness didn't last long, though. Out of nowhere a series of slicing, sharp pains crippled me. I could not walk, the pain only worsened upon movement.

I tried to sit on a heating pad, but the sensation of a dozen knives slicing my internal self only worsened.

"Want me to take you to the hospital?" my mom asked me worriedly.

The expression on my face was frozen in sheer misery.

"Not yet," I said stubbornly as I attempted to stand up and fight through the torturous pain.

Finally, I looked at my mother with tears in my eyes.

"Let's go," I muttered, "I think it ruptured!"

Each bump in the pavement on the way to the hospital tormented me. The pain was like nothing else I had ever faced before. It was three o'clock in the afternoon, and I now laid on a bed at the local ER.

A middle-aged man with a husky build, short brown hair and glasses opened the curtain to my room abruptly. A young intern followed behind him, although she never once spoke a word.

I explained to the doctor how much pain I was in and I told him of my recent ovarian cyst. Instead of listening to me though, he began to perform a series of unnecessary tests.

He returned to my room hours later with an odd expression on his face.

"Is it okay with you if I discuss your medical information in front of your mother?" the doctor asked.

I looked to my mother before looking back at him.

"Yes!" I responded with sincerity.

"Are you sure?" he asked again.

"Yes!" I said once more.

"Are you pregnant?"

"No."

"Okay..." he began with a sigh "are you sure about that?"

"Yes!"

"You are sure?"

"Yes, I'm sure!"

The doctor looked at me over his glasses.

"...Well, your urine test came back, and you are pregnant."

He stared at me and waited for me to react, as though I was supposed to fall out of bed in disappointment—or jump out of bed in celebration.

I could sense the judgement in the doctor's tone. He painted me out to be a reckless teenager full of lies.

I looked at him and laughed.

"No, I'm not. You are joking with me," I said with a smile, hoping to melt his frozen expression and cold stares.

He shook his head slowly, "We don't joke about these things around here."

I looked at his disappointed face and I shrugged my shoulders.

"Well, I'm not!" I said to him with a serious tone.

Of course I wasn't. I was seventeen years old, sick with a chronic illness and had a limited social life. I wouldn't lie to him, plus I very clearly told the doctor that I was here for a cyst that I believed ruptured.

"Well our tests don't lie," he said as he began to ask more and more uncomfortable questions.

Finally, my mother chimed in.

"She's not pregnant. She's really not. Your test is wrong," she told him.

The doctor looked at my mother blankly, seemingly unwilling to accept our responses.

Before long I found myself in the middle of the crossfire as my mom and the doctor fought over whether another human was growing inside of my body. I knew what was in my body—and it wasn't a baby—it was a cyst. I told the doctor this, but he refused to listen.

"Our test says that she is pregnant," he repeated.

"Nope, nope, nope! Retake the test. It's wrong," my mother said as she interrupted the repetitive doctor.

I'm not sure how, but God equipped mothers with so many different tools. Not only could my mom be quiet, gentle, and sweet, but when provoked she could make a stubborn, grown man with a strong, cemented opinion, walk out the door of my hospital room and recheck my test results.

I looked at my mother as she watched the doctor pull the curtain and silently leave my hospital room. She didn't even look at me. She had her angry mother bear mask on, and nobody was going to mess with her, or her cub.

The doctor returned minutes later, dragging his pride ten feet behind him.

"I apologize for that, I rechecked the test and it appears you are not pregnant after all."

He attempted to come up with an explanation for my test results gone wrong, but my mind zoned out. Whether my urine sample was mixed up with someone else's, or my urine results showed a false positive due to my cyst, it didn't matter to me. All that I could think of was how rude this doctor acted by not listening to me. As a patient, I deserved to be listened to—no matter what my test revealed. I felt betrayed, and my faith in this doctor was unraveling.

I soon had a CT scan which showed my large ovarian cyst. The doctor read the results and instructed me to go home and rest. He believed I could manage fine with ibuprofen and a heating pad, but I knew for sure that wouldn't help my level of pain.

After the doctor left and my discharge from the hospital was nearing, my nurse soon came back into my room. I asked her for some pain medication prior to my discharge, hoping it would at least provide me with enough relief to walk to the car and manage at home.

The nurse returned filling a small syringe with a heavy drug. She explained to me how the medication worked, but what she didn't tell me was just how powerful this medication was.

I sat in a chair beside my hospital bed. I was almost ready to go home. The nurse stood over me as she hooked the syringe onto my IV and pushed the plunger. Within a millisecond, everything changed.

The whole hospital room was on an angle, it just kept tilting. Quickly my eyes closed, and I began falling out of my chair. My head and body attempted to compensate for the dizzying drug but couldn't.

My nurse caught my falling body and guided me into bed. I was becoming increasingly unaware. I could not speak — words and sentences just wouldn't form.

I broke down into tears. I couldn't feel anything, and — although I was relieved to not have any pain — I wasn't even sure I still had a body. I whimpered and cried as my ability to tolerate severe depersonalization and detachment became strained. I tried to fight the drug, but soon I couldn't, and it overtook me completely.

My mother rubbed my hand in a predictable pattern. It was clear that her gentle, sweet side had returned.

I laid there in my dark hospital room for hours. My nurse was remarkable, she brought me cold cloths to cover my aching eyes. I didn't ask for them — I couldn't ask for them — but somehow, she knew I needed them.

I laid there unable to speak, but this fact bothered me less and less as the drug worked through my system. It seemed that the world didn't matter anymore. I was lying in a hospital bed, but I didn't know that — I could have been lying in the middle of a railroad, quite frankly, I didn't care. My body didn't feel like anything, I simply couldn't feel it.

My favorite pop song at the time, "Uptown Funk" by Mark Ronson featuring Bruno Mars, kept being played on the television in my room. Although I was out of it and struggled to speak, I laid in my bed and danced. Every time the song came on my body broke out in a random, jolting rhythm.

It was one of the only ways I felt I could communicate with my mom. As strange as it seems, I couldn't dance at any other time. I was too loopy and exhausted, I could barely even move—at least not until that song played.

Around three o'clock in the morning, my nurse walked into my room and woke me up. I had fallen into a very deep sleep. When I awoke, I was so happy and refreshed.

My nurse helped me stand up, but my balance was very off. My legs felt like they were way out at my sides, which made me prone to falling. I walked like a cowboy with giant leather chaps.

My nurse helped me into a wheelchair and wheeled me outside to my mom's car. She told me that the medication she gave me—Dilaudid—was something I shouldn't take again. She had a similar reaction to the medication when she was given it before, which is why she knew how to help me through the odd side effects so well.

"I had an ovarian cyst before too," my nurse said from behind me as she wheeled me outside, "they actually thought it was my appendix because it was on my right side. So, they removed my appendix then they realized it wasn't that at all, so I had to have a whole new surgery."

"Oh my goodness… that's awful…" I responded through my slow, slurred speech.

My nurse knew my pain firsthand.

The drive home was odd. The streets were empty, but as strange as it seems, I began to crave the nightlife. I was so awake and alive. Even though I could hardly walk a straight line, I couldn't feel my cyst anymore. I still could barely feel my body —I felt so good I just wanted to celebrate.

I chatted up a storm the whole ride home. I don't even remember anything I said.

Once I got home, I walked into my living room with my legs way out at my sides. As soon as I landed in the recliner, I fell right back to sleep. I slept like a rock.

As I opened my eyelids the next morning, I realized the pain from my cyst had returned, but this time it was coated with nausea.

I spent the entire summer day on the couch with a heating pad draped over my lower abdomen. Food was not appetizing today, and neither was water. The pain that once overtook my left side, now also overtook my right side directly below my ribs. Every position was uncomfortable, and pain medication barely brushed the surface of my pain.

By the time the evening rolled around, and my family was ready to settle down for dinner, my heart rate was well into the triple digits. I was out of breath, in excruciating pain, and I was certain I was dying.

My mom began to walk with me upstairs so that she could help me in the shower. As I was walking though, I grew upset. I didn't feel good—I told her that. But my mom had heard me mutter those words all too often in the past that she was not fully grasping that this time, I *really* meant it.

I turned to her with the same cemented look of pain I had the day before. Through my exhausted, air-hungry voice I muttered,

"I need to go to the doctor."

Getting into the car proved to be a difficult feat. I ever so slowly lifted my heavy legs and swung my body into the passenger seat of the car. Severe pain accompanied my every movement.

My parents and I were now headed to the doctor's office in town. Every bump in the road made me jolt up in agony.

"Please don't go over bumps!" I shouted to my parents in agony as I awkwardly sat in the car, unable to touch my painful stomach.

I laid on the exam table at the clinic with a heart rate monitor on my finger and a blood pressure cuff on my arm. The doctor hovered over my ailing body and reached out to touch my abdomen.

"Ah!" I screamed as tears immediately filled my eyes and I pushed the doctor's arm away, "Please don't touch me!" I cried.

The doctor backed up nervously before looking into my parents' eyes and dishing them dollops of concern.

My blood pressure was low, and my heart rate was around 150bpm as I rested on the exam table. It was clear by my increasing heart rate that my body was in severe pain. The doctor told me to go to the ER immediately—she believed my cyst had ruptured, and I needed medical attention right away.

I loaded back into my parents' car and soon arrived at the local ER—the same one I had just been discharged from less than twenty-four hours prior.

I sat in the waiting room fading from all existence. I was so dehydrated that I felt like I was hardly conscious. I could barely breathe. My heart rate was so high, and my body was so exhausted. I sat like a puffed-up old hen. My eyes closed as I continually faded from consciousness. I attempted desperately to inform my parents of my distant state, but I was so oxygen deprived that I could hardly speak.

Soon—after what seemed like an intense communication struggle—my father caught on to my plea and he rushed out of the ER doors.

He returned with a giant bottle of Gatorade and a straw. I drank the Gatorade as though it was my only lifeline. It provided very little relief, despite me drinking nearly half the bottle. The words of the miserable triage nurse from days prior echoed through my fading mind.

"You're not supposed to go to the bathroom, eat or drink if you are in the ER for abdominal pain!"

I took another sip of my Gatorade and continued to quickly slip away. I grabbed my mom's shoulder,

"We have to leave!" I instructed her.

I opened my eyes and looked at my dad with the most desperate look I could muster.

I continued to slip away with each passing minute. I grew more and more agitated as time ticked by and my connection to consciousness continued to fray. At this point, I didn't even care who else in the waiting room could hear me, I needed help.

"Please! Listen to me, I feel so bad!" I began to cry.

My mom asked the receptionist how long we would be waiting. The wait at this hospital was a couple of hours out, and I hadn't even seen a triage nurse yet. There was no way I could wait any longer.

"Let's go," my dad said as he began to head for the parking lot.

I followed behind him ever so slowly.

My body was hunched over like a ninety-year-old, my arms tucked gently at my sides. Each step I took was as light footed as possible as to not cause further pain. People around me stared, but quite frankly I didn't care. I didn't know where we were headed, all I knew was that I needed help, and I needed it yesterday.

I was now in the back seat of my dad's car. I was not even holding on to reality anymore. My body felt like it was giving up completely, but help was still at least an hour out. I don't even remember the ride to the hospital.

I sat in a waiting room of a new hospital, surrounded by little kids. I cowered on one end of a rounded leather seat as my entire body shook. My eyes stayed shut. I could feel my dad's presence to my left, and I rested my head on his shoulder. It took everything in me to communicate how I felt to him.

I couldn't wait any longer, and I told him that. My mother was sitting across from a triage nurse on the other side of the room. I could feel my dad get up from his seat abruptly. Suddenly someone took me by my arm.

"I feel like passing out," I mumbled, unable to keep my eyes open long enough to fully see the man holding on to me.

The mystery hospital worker supported a lot of my weight as I struggled to stand up. He guided my weak, half-awake body onto a scale.

"I think I'm going to pass out," I continued to warn him.

My legs were giving out, and things were escalating quickly. The man caught me as I nearly fell to the floor. He escorted me straight to a room where I laid on a bed with my eyes closed. My whole body trembled. I curled up in pain.

"Why am..." I tried to speak but the words wouldn't escape in time through my fading mind, "I don't get..." I attempted desperately to communicate how I felt, "why am I so out of it and tired?"

"You seem fine to me. I mean, you are talking," the man told me.

I was much too dazed to fight. I didn't know what I had to do or say to people for them to realize I was not fine. Everything I was experiencing was not normal, but I had zero energy to prove it. It seemed that the entire world was denying my obvious calls for help.

My body had blared all the internal alarms it could to warn me that something major was wrong. I could hear the alarms through my crippling pain, loss of appetite, nausea, and fatigue. Now though, the alarms were turning into mayday calls as sharp pain accompanied my every breath and my consciousness waned.

After sitting with me for a couple of minutes and gathering my information from my parents, the man disappeared down the hall. My body felt like it was in shock. I was so distant that I could hardly communicate. I was plummeting down the endless doom of unconsciousness.

Chapter Thirteen
Finding Strength from a Seagull

He whispered so softly inside her ear
"I am your greatest strength, release to me your fear"
She did just as He said, allowing herself to let go
All the pain and fear she kept, she released to Him very slow
She immediately felt more lifted, she felt so very strong
All her anxieties, fears, and obstacles were gone

— *"Release Your Fears" by Shayla Rose*

I COULD FEEL the cool liquid of an IV going through my arm. I was in a new room now, and ever so slowly I was becoming more aware.

A man wearing scrubs came into my room and pressed on my stomach.

"No! It hurts!" I cried and whimpered as I used all my strength to push him away. I had no manners, all I had was pain and instincts.

Soon a new doctor came in and, she too, pressed on my stomach. My body folded up in pain. I couldn't handle one more ounce of pressure on my tender abdomen. Just the slightest pressure made my already high pain level, skyrocket.
They wouldn't back off though. They both hovered over me and touched my stomach as I screamed, cried, and fought back. They were persistent and serious. Nothing I could do or say

would make them stop touching my excruciating abdomen. I felt helpless.

Everyone who pressed on my stomach wore the same face of dreadful concern. After what seemed like an eternity, they finally stopped touching me.

I asked for pain medication, "Please don't give me Dilaudid though. I don't react well to it," I told the man who just finished pressing on my stomach.

"Well we may not have a choice. There isn't a whole lot of pain management options."

I laid there worriedly. I didn't want to go through another dreadful drug experience, and this man didn't seem to take my concerns seriously.

A young nurse with a country twang came in and cared for me. She set me up with morphine and catered to all my needs. After spending much of the night waiting for test results and watching outdated sitcoms on the TV, the doctor returned.

"A nurse is going to come and get you and they are going to wheel you upstairs for an ultrasound, okay?

"Okay."

After being wheeled across the hospital, I now laid on my bed in a dark room with my parents to my left side. A woman sat in front of the nearby ultrasound machine. She was dressed up nicely—a far cry from scrubs and lab coats.

As I soon learned, it was now six o'clock in the morning. I spent the duration of my ultrasound pondering where the night went. You lose your perception of time quickly in a hospital setting, because after all, hospitals never sleep.

"Is your bladder full?" she asked me as she began to pour warm gel over my abdomen.

"I'm not sure."

I couldn't feel my bladder. My whole abdomen was in so much bloated discomfort, I could not tell.

She spent a longtime staring at the ultrasound monitor as she rolled the ultrasound wand across my sensitive belly. Soon, she called somebody on the phone and two other women crowded around the machine.

I laid on my bed for two hours and watched these three women distinguish each part of my stomach. It was very evident that they saw something. I listened to them as they seemed to speak a foreign language consisting of long, unrecognizable medical terms.

By this point my right side hurt worse than my left. I had a constant, sharp pain under my ribcage that got worse each time I took a breath.

"Oh yes your bladder is very full!" one of the women said eagerly.

"Really? I can't feel it," I said humorously.

I was wheeled back downstairs after the lengthy ultrasound concluded. The doctor returned to my room just as she was finishing up her shift.

"So, it looks like you have a large ovarian cyst on your left ovary that ruptured. You are free to go home though," she said to me in part, "unless you want to stay for observation."

I looked at her perplexed.

"But I'm just going to be in more pain again if I go home. I really think I should stay longer," I told her.

I was not willing to leave the hospital without some form of treatment. I knew something more had to be going on. I was in too much pain to be discharged. There was something seriously wrong and I wasn't going home until I felt better.

The doctor agreed to let me stay. She called around the hospital and found an empty room in the neurology unit for me.

The wheels on my bed unlocked with a kick. The hallways zoomed passed me. The elevator dinged. I slowly turned the corner to a large room with a big window. My bed was now locked into place.

"Hello, I'm Mike!" a young nurse with short dark hair, a stocky build and an excitable energy came into my room and introduced himself. He asked me what was going on, and we explained to him our long adventure.

We all knew I had a cyst, but because I hadn't gone to the bathroom in a couple of days people began to blame my pain for constipation. I was constipated, sure, but I also was hardly eating.

Mike excitedly offered me English muffins and peanut butter. English muffins were Mike's strong suit.

After eating my delicious breakfast, my parents looked at me, exhausted.

"We are going to go home for a while," my mother said, "but we will be back soon, okay?"

I was afraid to see them go at first. I had never been in the city all alone before. My parents were my best advocates and watching them leave made me feel vulnerable.

"She'll be fine, she's a big kid," Mike said to my parents as they began to grab their things.

After a quick hug and kiss, my parents were off.

My hospital room was so large, it was even larger now that I was alone. The floor was a shiny laminate. A large bathroom was right at the foot of my bed and a beautiful window was to my right. I wasn't sure what I had done to deserve such a cozy, private suite, but I sure wasn't complaining.

After my parents left the hospital, I fell asleep. I drifted right off into a comfortable snooze. I woke up to Mike touching my left arm as he attempted to check my blood pressure.

"Oops," Mike said as he saw my eyes open, "I didn't mean to wake you. Did you have a nice nap?"

"Yeah," I said with a yawn.

"You have a test in a half an hour, so rest up!"

Before long Mike returned with a wheelchair. He pushed me through the maze of the hospital so effortlessly. I could never understand how nurses knew exactly where to go, everything looked the same to me in this giant medical building.

117

He parked me right at the door of a small dark room. Two women arrived, and Mike spoke with them briefly before he helped guide me into a bed.

"I'll be back in a bit to pick you up!" he told me.

"Okay, thank you."

The two ultrasound technicians didn't speak much, they were very serious. They mainly spoke quietly amongst themselves—except of course when one of the women asked me an interesting question.

"How old are you honey, twelve?" one of the women asked me.

"No, I'm seventeen," I replied.

"Oh! I'm sorry," she responded with an embarrassed laughter, "you look so young."

I laid there and looked off at the wall paintings in front of me as the two women became fascinated with the ultrasound monitor.

After the test was finished, I went back into my wheelchair and waited. The two women left the room and I sat there alone. Mike was nowhere to be found, and I was worried. I didn't know where my room was—or where I was for that matter. My wheelchair was locked, and it hurt my abdomen too much to move. I was too dizzy to stand, so I sat there. Five minutes went by, ten minutes went by, and just as I was beginning to plot my grand hospital escape, Mike came around the corner.

I breathed a sigh of relief.

"All set?" Mike asked, "Sorry I'm late, how did it go?"

"Good I think!"

We chatted the whole way upstairs.

"Are you getting hungry? Do you want me to help you order lunch when we get back?"

"Um... I'm not really that hungry."

"Yeah, but you should eat something! How about an English muffin?"

"No..."

"Are you sure? You can have peanut butter again, like you did this morning."

"No, that's okay."

"How about soup?"

"Okay."

I wasn't hungry, but Mike was persuasive.

I sat up in my recliner and I waited for my soup to arrive. I wasn't the least bit hungry, I was still so bloated and uncomfortable.

A woman pushed a shiny metal cart down the hallway and opened the door to my large hospital room. She placed my soup on my small side table with a smile,

"Here's your soup, enjoy!"

I stared at it. I could smell the steam of the chicken broth and my mind echoed with Mike's words.

"You have to eat something."

I reached for the small package of oyster crackers that teetered on top of my soup bowl and opened it, but just as I was thinking of putting a cracker in my mouth, a tall man wearing blue scrubs rushed in my room.

"Hi, are you Shayla?" the man said eagerly.

"Yes," I responded, attempting to piece together his stressed body language and serious tone.

"Have you eaten your soup yet?"

"No."

"Good!" he said with relief, "You won't be needing that!"

He moved my soup out of reach before sitting down across from me. My eyes followed my soup as it slid away from me as quickly as it had arrived.

"So, my name is Dr. Willis and I am one of the surgeons here. It looks like you are going to need surgery."

I looked at him puzzled.

The surgeon explained to me that my recent ultrasound results were not good. There was a high chance that my large cyst caused me to have an ovarian torsion—where the ovary wraps itself around the fallopian tube and cuts off the blood supply to the ovary. In the case of an ovarian torsion, the ovary sometimes needs to be removed completely, while other times it can be saved.

Mike ran into my room at what seemed like one hundred miles an hour.

"Don't eat anything!" he shouted.

A look of relief washed over his face as he realized my soup bowl was out of arms reach.

"I already told her," the surgeon explained with a half-smile.

"Oh good! Phew! I just told her she could have soup." Mike breathed heavily as he tried to recover from his frantic run around the neurology unit.

"When do I have to have surgery?" I asked the surgeon worriedly.

"Now."

After failing to convince the surgeon that I did not need surgery, I asked him if we could at least wait for my parents to return. The surgeon agreed to wait for my parents as he began to get things into place, but he didn't seem comfortable with waiting too long. I called my mom on the phone, and—despite being caught in traffic—she managed to walk into my hospital room right as Dr. Willis returned.

Dr. Willis handed me paperwork and quickly discussed the surgery with my mother. I signed a couple of documents and then Mike and another nurse arrived. They unlocked my bed and wheeled me down a series of hallways before parking me in the pre-operating room.

I was nervous, I had never had surgery before. Everything was happening so fast, I barely had enough time to think.

"Good luck!" Mike said as he walked away.

To my right stood my anesthesiologist—a middle aged woman with a gentle, soothing voice. She explained to me what I should expect and prepared the magical concoction of drugs that would shut my lights out.

I gave my mom an emotional hug, and I prayed to God in desperation as I quickly fell to sleep with the push of a plunger. Moments later I woke up.

"Why are you strapping me down?" I asked the two women who were carrying me.

Beneath my body was a hard table with red Velcro straps. I didn't understand what was going on, but the survival instinct in me was ready to fight. I thought I was being kidnapped by two strangers, and I was mad. Except, I didn't know what to do about it.

"It's okay honey, these straps are just to keep you safe. You're okay, just go back to sleep," the anesthesiologist said in her familiar gentle tone as she grabbed my leg and strapped it to the table.

"Oh, okay then," I said as I closed my eyes, willing to accept the answers from my gentle kidnappers who were dressed in strange hats and masks.

I could hear the two women laughing, so I laughed too. Then, I fell asleep.

I woke up with a mask over my face and my anesthesiologist sitting at my right side. I threw up as soon as I woke up. My shoulders ached so badly. I was nauseated, and my lower stomach felt sore. I spent a while piecing everything together. My mom came over to me in the recovery room and held my hand.

My surgery went well, and I was able to keep both of my ovaries. My intense pain that I experienced was likely caused from when my cyst ruptured. It ruptured against a blood vessel and blood filled up my abdomen. My right side below my ribs hurt because the blood from the rupture was pooling there and irritating my liver. During surgery, a very large amount of blood and fluid was drained from my abdomen.

Right after waking up from surgery, I was wheeled into the elevator. I was still in a groggy state, but eventually I woke up to a new room with a new nurse.

My nurse's name was Anne and she was barely even five feet tall. She had a caring, gentle presence and she was very pregnant.

It was now around eight o'clock at night. My shoulders and neck were in so much pain from the air that was pumped into my stomach during surgery. Most of the night was spent with Anne repositioning me in bed, loading my neck up with ice packs and giving me shoulder massages.

In the wee hours of the morning, I woke up to Anne checking on me.

"Are you okay?" Anne whispered as she walked to my bedside and placed a gentle hand on my arm.

"I have to go pee," I whispered back, trying not to wake my mom who was sleeping beside me in a hospital recliner.

"Okay, hold on."

She helped me out of bed and followed slowly behind me with my IV tower. We got into the bathroom and Anne stood across from me. My bladder felt so full, but once I sat down nothing came out.

"I just can't go," I told Anne.

"Really? Do you want me to leave, maybe that will help?"

"No, that's okay. Let me keep trying."

After several minutes went by, I still couldn't go. I began carefully laughing—trying not to cause further pain.

"Your bladder is still sleeping from the surgery!" she told me, "Hold on, I'll be right back."

Anne left while another nurse stayed with me. She returned with a small container of peppermint.

"Smell this," she told me as she placed the peppermint in my hand and turned the sink faucet on.

After a couple of whiffs of peppermint and several eager attempts, I peed.

"Good job!" Anne cheered.

We both quietly laughed at the humorous situation before Anne returned me safely to my bed.

Around nine o'clock in the morning, Anne said a sad goodbye to me. Her shift was over, and I couldn't stop crying. I'm not sure if it was the medications I was on or what, but I began to get very emotional. I very quickly bonded with Anne, and seeing her go felt like losing a lifelong friend.

A new nurse took her place, but my kind treatment was beginning to fade.

My roommate was a teenage girl recovering from back surgery. My heart ached for her as she screamed and cried in pain for the entire day.

I was discharged from the hospital the day after my surgery. I cried as I left the hospital, and I'm not sure why. I wanted to leave, but at the same time I was scared to. The hospital staff were kind to me, and I only hoped I could cope okay on my own.

The next day, I sat in my mom's car in the parking lot of our local drug store. My mom went in the store to pick up a nausea medication for me. I was so depersonalized and exhausted. I hadn't had much to drink at all due to the nausea and pain that my recovering body was undergoing, so I was left feeling very out of it. I felt like I was dying, I was so weak.

As I sat there all alone, I prayed to God in desperation. I asked Him to help me recover, and to give me the strength I needed to continue.

As I looked out the car window for a sign of hope, I saw a beautiful white seagull fly across the backdrop of several large pine trees. I wasn't sure why the sight of this seagull comforted me so much, but it did. The seagull relieved me of my worries. I stared at its gracefulness as it glided across the sky and I instantly felt my fears lift away. Despite my intense symptoms, seeing this faithful seagull reassured me that I could go on.

After a couple weeks of recovery, I was back to normal. Only a small scar was left to forever remind me of my agonizing adventure.

Chapter Fourteen
Just a Dizzy Server

I had a suitcase made from leather
Its storage seemed to go on forever
In my suitcase I tossed all my distress
All my symptoms I refused to address
But it compiled over time and the lid wouldn't shut
Surely by now I was in a deep rut
I tried to sit on top, with my weight on the lid
But out poured all my struggles I had always hid
The time was short before I noticed the stress on its seams
It was clear I was living very outside of my means

— *"The Suitcase" by Shayla Rose*

I THOUGHT I WAS making it to the point of being normal again. I upheld a baseline of symptoms that were relatively manageable. I still experienced lightheadedness, brain fog, headaches, fatigue, shortness of breath, tachycardia, vomiting, and more, but I was able to know my limits and tried my hardest not to exceed them.

I wanted my life back more than I ever wanted it before. The older I became the more that my dependence ate at me. I spent most of my time as an eighteen-year-old sitting at home, hoping. I hoped for many things from the confines of my living room, but the thing I hoped for most was independence. I wanted freedom from the jail cell of my illness.

Every week I sat in the passenger seat of my mother's car, watching the scenery go by my window as we rode around town running errands. I stared out the car window looking desperately for something to rescue me from the choke hold of my illness and from the dim light of my inevitable depression. I wanted to be a part of something much greater than myself. I wanted to leave more than just my footprints in my small town. I wasn't living, even though I was alive. Each night when I laid down to sleep, the lingering desire to find something more taunted me.

Eventually, my intense longing was over. I found precisely what I was looking for, and it was closer than I thought.

A new building stood in town, towering over all the other buildings it stood beside. It was so tall, and its architecture was so impressive, I couldn't help but wonder what it would hold. I watched its slow progression over the course of many months.

Men were suspended from its roof as they pounded nails into its siding. They worked tirelessly constructing this large mysterious building, and soon, after much anticipation, the time-lapse of its development was complete.

I stood in the doorway and slowly removed my polarized sunglasses from my face. The smell of new beginnings filled the air of the empty building. The carpet beneath my shoes held not one stain and the freshly painted walls were nearly still tacky.

Around me were many workers. Some unboxed furniture while others installed light fixtures. I breathed in the fresh smell of renovation and I savored the sight of one person's dream being birthed. As I stood there embracing the inside of this large building, my once-nervous butterflies flew in anxious excitement. I finally found what I was looking for.

"You can start orientation next week!" the job interviewer told me, in the middle of the chaos that surrounded us, "Does that work for you?"

"Yes!" I said excitedly.

I couldn't hold back my enthusiasm. Soon my dimples showed themselves and the fluttering butterflies in my stomach turned into floating confetti. I could hardly wait to begin working.

Orientation nearly killed me. After an eight-hour long day of being taught how to work in a culinary setting, I sat in my mother's car chugging water like a drunk looking to sober up. The world around me was so hard to comprehend. I felt like I was watching my life through the bottom of a glass—everything was so distant. I was so removed from the world, and so removed from my body. The energy I lost during eight hours of grueling orientation nearly sent me to the hospital. I cried—in defeat and fear, and I began to question my ability to take on this new job.

Despite orientation sending me to my knees, I was not about to give up. I was hired as a server in the dining room of a newly polished retirement home. In my white buttoned shirt and my black slacks, I balanced trays and bussed tables. I took my new job as a privilege, and I worked tirelessly every shift to keep it.

I didn't tell anyone that I was sick—I never even told my boss. I held a fear that my illness would make others underestimate me. I worried that, if my health was disclosed, the doors to my beloved job would close. Too much had been taken away from me, and I didn't want my new job to be added to the list. It wasn't until I couldn't hide my illness a day longer that I realized my secret truth was already known.

As much as I tried, no amount of stubbornness could keep my illness away. I began to wake up every morning searching for more oxygen. My heart rate climbed overnight, and by morning it was already well into the triple digits. My need for food and hydration was dire when I awoke. I felt so awful every morning that I couldn't even carry on a conversation with my family members until after I ate breakfast. I simply had no air, no patience, and no energy. Despite these rough mornings, I continued working each afternoon.

One afternoon during the lunch shift, the quaint dining room busted at its seams. Thirty hungry people arrived for lunch and me and my coworker were firing from all cylinders.

"Do you have them?" she asked me, referring to the next three people entering the dining room, her hands juggling coffee cups and place settings.

"Yes!" I said helpfully, as I carried menus and water to the new arrivals.

An hour or two into my lunch shift, my energy levels bottomed out. Walking to the kitchen and back to the dining room felt like the length of a football field. My legs felt like they were weighed down with lead weights, pulling me closer and closer to the floor.

"You don't feel good, do you?" my coworker asked me as I slowly wiped down the counters at the end of the lunch rush.

"No, I don't feel good. I have low blood pressure," I pointed out, unwilling to dive into the details of my past.

"You look like you have low blood sugar," she said, "I had low blood sugar when I was your age. Are you sure you don't have hypoglycemia?"

Hypoglycemia?

I had never heard of hypoglycemia before, so I doubt I had it.

"No, I don't think so. I just feel like I'm in a dream most of the time," I responded.

"Yeah, you feel really dazed, right? And tired?"

"Yeah."

"Sounds like hypoglycemia to me," she insisted.

"I have to rest for a minute," I told her as I took a chair in the dining room and placed peanut butter coated crackers in my mouth.

It was interesting to me that my coworker could see through my pale, fading composure, that my blood sugar was depleted. I wasn't sure if she was right, but the way that food revived me had me seriously wondering.

I'm so dizzy, please pick me up.

I texted my parents desperately.

I left that day feeling as though I was at deaths door. I looked to food to save me as I traveled home in my father's car. I was so overworked that the roads and houses that we passed by on the way home looked oddly unfamiliar to me. I was hardly able to talk due to my intense feeling of nearly losing consciousness. I couldn't get home quick enough.

I battled fiercely to feel better and make my way out of the thick fog. I felt so overworked, but no matter what I did I could not find the relief I was longing for. After throwing every morsel of food I could find into my mouth, I slept on the couch for the remainder of the afternoon.

"I think I need to go to the doctor," I said to my father the next morning, "will you please take me to the clinic?"

He started up his truck and the entire nearby woodland shook. The squirrels lost their acorns from their grip and the trees dropped their leaves as my father's locomotive-sounding pickup truck roared.

I hopped inside his truck and cried as the clinic came closer.

"Can we just go home?" I asked my dad.

"What? Why?"

"I hate this place. I don't even want to go in. I come here so often," I whimpered to my dad from the parking lot of the clinic.

It seemed like my trips to the local clinic were becoming so frequent. I could sense by the stares I received from the full-time nurse at the clinic that she judged me. She thought I was a hypochondriac, and the more I visited the clinic, the more difficult it became for me to even believe myself.

"C'mon Shay, it's fine," my dad attempted to reassure me.

"No dad, you don't get it! The nurse in here judges me. I can't keep doing this to myself! I'm such an idiot. Why do I even come here, I'm just wasting everyone's time!"

"So, what do you want me to do?"

"Go home, I just can't go in there!"

"What if I go in first?"

"I don't know," I broke down in tears. My dad handed me a tissue out of his shirt pocket, he always had a convenient stack of them handy.

"Come on, let's go," my dad guided me out of the truck by my arm and held my hand as we walked inside.

I sat in the waiting room with my father by my side. I was hoping beyond hope that the dreadful nurse had taken the day off, but that was sadly not the case. My dad tried to initiate small talk with her as she called me into the exam room and checked my vitals, but she was not at all friendly.

After a short wait, I was sitting across from the doctor, a middle-aged man with a comforting tone.

"I wake up every morning short of breath. I also have to eat really frequently or else I feel like passing out," I told him the entirety of my symptoms.

"She's been to doctors before and they never find anything, but you can tell that she doesn't feel good. She looks so pale sometimes, like the life is sucked right out of her," my dad told the doctor, nearly begging him for answers.

An EKG was ordered, as was a chest x-ray and a blood sugar check. After waiting only a short time, the doctor came back in and sat on his swiveling stool.

"Well the EKG came back abnormal," he began, "so I think you need to set up an appointment with a cardiologist. Also, your blood sugar today is low, you may have hypoglycemia."

After a few minutes of conversation, my dad and I left the office with an appointment card to a new cardiologist, and a pending diagnosis first spotted from a coworker.

A couple of weeks later I sat in the office of my new cardiologist. My stomach rolled, and a heavy feeling of nausea lingered. I was dehydrated and exhausted from throwing up the entire night before—a new occurrence that was becoming more frequent.

"I have to go to the bathroom!" I whispered to my mom who gave me an uneasy look, "I'll be fast!" I promised her as I slowly got out of my seat and maneuvered my way through the hallway to the bathroom.

It was hard to see straight as I fought through blacking out every time I stood. After a bout of unavoidable diarrhea, I finally made it back to the exam room just in time to meet my new doctor.

He reviewed my recent EKG and ordered a full cardiac workup for me, including a twenty-four-hour heart monitor, an echocardiogram, and an appointment for a stress test. All these tests came back normal. Still, I fought with being chronically out of breath.

I later followed up with my primary care doctor who confirmed my hypoglycemia diagnosis.

I continued to go to work every evening like clockwork. I enjoyed my job immensely and I was now a daily part of the lives of the retirement home residents. Every time I wasn't at work, work was all I could think about.

I stood in the kitchen of the retirement home one afternoon on my day off.

"Shayla!" my boss said as he peered at me over the kitchen line, "You aren't supposed to be here today!"

"I just can't leave this place!" I jokingly shouted back to him, waiting for him to finish cooking.

We joked about how much I loved my job, and how often I was there.

"I'm here because you gave me three days off! I want to work!" I told him with a serious tone and a smiling face, "I can't be home for three days!"

He changed the schedule around and laughed at my devotion. I walked out happy, knowing I could spend an extra shift doing what I loved.

My passion for my job was unlike any other. I practically lived at work, and when I wasn't there, I counted down the hours until I was. I was a hard worker, until my illness once again reared its ugly head.

Soon my lower back hurt and—after a quick visit to the clinic—it was discovered that I had a bad urinary tract infection that was beginning to travel to my kidneys. After a round of antibiotics, which left my stomach an uneasy disaster, I went back to the clinic one afternoon just before work.

"Wow! Your blood pressure is low!" the nurse said, concerned, "Do you feel alright?" he wondered.

"Yes, I'm always dizzy," I told him as I attempted to piece together my low numbers. I stared at the tiled floor and bit my lip, questioning if I really was okay.

That evening at four o'clock, my mother dropped me off at work. I was excited for my shift, despite having lingering fatigue I just couldn't shake.

"Hey! I saw your grandson the other day!" I greeted two of the residents as they slowly wobbled down to the dining room behind their metal walkers.

They started to speak to me, but my hearing began to fade, and my dwindling concentration left me stranded mid-conversation. My vision blurred, my body swayed, and my knees began to buckle. I hurried into the kitchen, as a pounding pulse overtook my head.

"I'm about to faint!" I yelled to my coworker as I laid out on the floor and attempted to regain my senses.

"Oh okay," she said, only slightly startled.

I asked her desperately to retrieve my snack bag from the nearby cupboard and I began guzzling fluids and every morsel of salt and protein my bag contained.
    I tried to stand, but the sensation of passing out wouldn't let me go. Still, despite my body showing every possible sign of POTS, I blamed myself.

I'm such an idiot, it's all in my head.

I attempted to feed myself the same diagnosis so many people had tried to feed me. Being unable to understand why I felt so many symptoms at once, I attempted to convince myself I was suffering from an anxiety-derived illness.

"You're a fighter! I like that," my coworker said to me as she passed through the serving area juggling guest checks and trays of food.

"Oh..." I said with a half-grin, "thank you. I'm sort of used to it."

"Yeah," she said as she stared at me for a couple of seconds and nodded her head.

I called my parents and told them I needed them to pick me up from work early. I walked out of work with the aid of a coworker to the safety of my dad's car.

I went to sleep that night brushing off my flare. I was hoping it was a scary fluke. The next day, like clockwork, I put on my black slacks and fastened my bowtie. I wasn't going down that easy, it was going to take much more than one episode to make me give up.

I hid my symptoms from those around me. I tried desperately to brush my ailments under the rug, in hopes that I could fake myself into being healthy. It didn't work though, and soon I was a server who couldn't stand — a waitress who couldn't balance a tray.

Fatigue overtook me, and I struggled to even keep my eyes open. I was operating in a deep fog of detachment, and it scared me. Memorizing orders became impossible, but writing was just as taxing. I became the kitchen's weakest link in a matter of days.

My near fainting spells repeated themselves every shift. It got to the point that, for the safety of myself and others, I could no longer work.

"I don't want to leave. We are so shorthanded!" I told my boss with tears in my eyes as I laid on the serving room floor, trying to avoid passing out.

"You need to take care of you! You can always come back," my boss muttered, laughing at my devotion.

As I laid on the cold hardwood floor in the serving area of my beloved job, I knew it was the end. I knew that leaving was not as simple as walking out and coming back when I felt better. I knew that in the moment I left, I was turning the page back into my illness. I didn't want to go back into the world of sickness. I fought so hard to not let go, but I had no choice. My illness claimed me again.

"I just need a couple weeks off!" I told my boss as I bumped into the ice cream chest on my way out the door, "Just a couple! I'll be back when I feel better."

"Take your time," my boss told me, laughing and mumbling a compliment under his breath.

The rope that tethered me to my newly-found happiness and independence frayed. I watched each delicate piece of rope unwind until a mere fiber remained. I closed my eyes and loosened my grip, choosing it to be better to fall with dignity and grace than the alternative.

Chapter Fifteen
Welcome Back to Chronic Illness, Love

She faced it for years, that deep feeling of deception
It became profound, each night in that mirrored reflection
Where did she go wrong? How is she here?
Was it her own fault? Her own subconscious fear?
The mirrored reflection that stood blinking back
Haunted her, taunted her, and took her off track
At first just a trickle, now a steady stream
The emotions so heavy, she let out a scream
It was more than a moan but less than a yell
Just in that moment, she fell
Her cold palms laid on the even colder tile
Her taunting troubles laid beside her in a pile
She nearly drowned from the constant current of tears
That deep feeling of deception, she faced it for years

— *"Mirrors of Deception" by Shayla Rose*

I WALKED THROUGH the front door of my house and shook my head. Defeat overcame me as I relived each moment of my last shift. I laid on the couch with my feet propped up on an extra cushion and stared at the white ceiling above me. I laid there in reflection, unable to escape the cold grip of my illness.

I felt like I was on a boat during rough seas. I could feel myself moving and slowly falling, as though I was descending off the edge of the couch. As time went on the speed of my fall increased. Except, I did not move an inch.

"Time for supper!" my mom shouted, her voice perking up every creature within a one-mile radius.

I sat at the dinner table and lined empty chairs on either side of me, caging myself in. Somehow, in my dizzy head, I felt that the back of the chairs would prevent me from falling out of my seat.

I began eating—one bite was chewed and swallowed, another bite was chewed and swallowed, until I forgot how to swallow completely.

I sat there, surrounded by my family at the dinner table, with stubborn mashed potatoes threatening my windpipe. I sipped some milk and ever so slowly tricked my throat into swallowing. Before long, I collapsed my head into my palms in defeat.

"I can't do this!" I muttered, with my elbows on the table in frustration.

My mom took my plate.

"C'mon," she ordered, "you can go eat in the living room."

She set me up in the recliner, elevated my legs with pillows, and passed me my dinner.

Upright posture was now too symptom provoking to handle. The recliner became my landing zone, and this fact terrified me.

That night I sat on my old plastic stool in the shower, too weak to stand.

"Can you please help me wash my hair?" I asked my mom, too dizzy to keep my arms above my head.

"Yes," she responded.

"I'm getting worse again," I told my mom as she lathered my hair with conditioner.

"Oh, please don't say that," she responded, as we both dwelled on my worsening health and feared the thought of me becoming bedridden again.

I sat there, hoping beyond hope that the doomed feeling within me—the instinctual hint telling me I was getting sicker—was wrong.

As my health began to remove me again from the outside world, a deep feeling of sorrow sunk inside my chest. So many things had been taken away from me in the past few years of my life. My life was filled with missed opportunities and abandoned friendships because of my illness. Just as I gained my footing once more—after years of fighting for it—my happiness dangled before my face. I reached out to grab the happiness and health I worked for as it teased my fingertips, but at the last second it was yanked away.

Just as we feared, I soon became too ill to function. I was draped in a heavy coat of lightheadedness and vertigo. I could no longer walk the length of my house without nearly collapsing. I was so fatigued and depersonalized that I could no longer go through the day without taking several naps. I was too dizzy to sit upright, and too lightheaded to brush my teeth without being supported.

I was confined to the recliner all day long. My world became smaller and smaller by the day. Each day more and more of my abilities and independence faded. I was struggling to adapt to my new normal of confinement.

My isolation went unnoticed to many people, aside from my coworkers or close family that were a part of my daily routine. Most did not realize how sick I became.

I went to the gastroenterologist for a follow-up appointment for my acid reflux, vomiting, and irritable bowel syndrome weeks later.

I was so sick that leaving the house to go to the doctor's office was a great challenge. I dreaded leaving my recliner, let alone the house.

The exam table in the exam room was so short that I could not lay down. My legs hung off its edge and I quickly became uncomfortable as my body swayed side to side. I was knocked around by dizziness, and I feared I would fall off the exam table completely. Soon I sat in a nearby chair and elevated my legs high on the exam table, hoping to avoid passing out. I hid my face from the fluorescent lights above me and I tried desperately to balance and calm my swaying body.

"Hey!" my doctor greeted my mother and I as he walked through the door.

He watched me in worry as I struggled to keep my eyes open. I fidgeted in my chair, unable to escape the grip of my illness.

"I know she gets dizzy, but because her symptoms are worsening, you guys should follow up with her primary care physician. This isn't safe. She could fall, she shouldn't even be in the kitchen preparing food or anything. This just isn't safe," my doctor advised us with appropriate concern as we told him about my recent relapse in symptoms.

I'm not even sure if we discussed my acid reflux or IBS at this appointment. My doctor was so concerned about the progression of my POTS that he could barely focus on much else. We left the gastroenterologist that day and soon scheduled an appointment with my primary care doctor.

I was becoming so much worse in such a short amount of time. I went from working on my feet every day and bringing people their dinner, to not being able to stand long enough to pour myself a glass of water. I became so dependent on my family for every task. I got progressively worse and there was no end to my deterioration in sight. I couldn't even go to the bathroom alone anymore, or else I would fall right off the toilet. I was bound to our small, quiet living room and I couldn't understand why.

"Your blood pressure is low!" my primary care doctor told me as I glanced at her through my polarized sunglasses, hoping to block out the light and in turn keep my eyes open longer, "Your heart is working very hard to compensate for your low blood pressure. I can give you something for that, hold on a minute," my passionate doctor left the exam room briefly before returning.

She decided to start me on a corticosteroid called fludrocortisone, the same medication I was prescribed in the early days of my illness.

After having my cortisol levels checked, I took the medication. Over time I experienced less tachycardia and my blood pressure became more regulated, however, my other debilitating symptoms remained.

It was becoming clearer by the day that I wasn't getting much better. My father held on to me one afternoon as I walked to the kitchen to make myself a sandwich.

"Don't let go!" I pleaded, knowing that as soon as his strong, supporting grip left me I would be swallowed by a dizzy wave and caught by the hard ground.

"I have to go to the bathroom," I told my mom frequently, as I got up from the recliner and attempted to walk a straight line to the bathroom.

She rushed to my aid several times every day as my legs took me in the opposite direction and I nearly walked in to the entertainment center or the fireplace.

Requiring help with every task began to burden my family. My parents occasionally grew frustrated at my dependency.

"You have separation anxiety! Why can't you go to the bathroom alone!" my dad shouted at me in a fit of frustration one day as I asked my mom to stand with me in the bathroom.

Tears poured from my tired, dizzy eyes as I continued to question my authenticity.

Am I really suffering from separation anxiety?!

There was very little that I could do to improve my health. Being in the midst of a chronic illness episode is like being caught in a bad windstorm. As the wind blows against you, you have nowhere to turn. You cannot fight against the powerful windstorm—it's simply too strong. For days, weeks, months or years—you wait for the wind to change direction, even if only briefly, so that you can finally continue on your life as normal.

My new normal was becoming abnormal, even to me. Every day I cried in grief, fear, and disappointment. I couldn't understand why I settled into such a bad rut of symptoms. Every few weeks I was waking up in the middle of the night to vomit. My energy levels were bottomed out—I couldn't even lift a table lamp without napping immediately after. The lightweight, ten-pound porcelain lamp felt like the equivalent of lifting another human. I was spending more hours asleep than awake.

My dizziness was off the charts, my depersonalization made life itself frightening. I was not even half the person I was a couple of months prior.

I stared at a basket of laundry one afternoon, in the early days of March as I sat in my recliner. I twiddled my thumbs as the pile of unfolded laundry taunted me.

You won't get better unless you exercise! Get up and fold that laundry!

My mind talked to my body like a drill sergeant.

I reluctantly stood up from the safe haven of my recliner. My vision began to darken as I attempted to acclimate to the gravity pulling on my tired circulatory system. My eyelids were heavy, and my mind was filled with brain fog. I felt like I was walking on uneven terrain as I walked five feet to the basket of laundry sitting on the accompanying couch.

I took out one towel from the laundry basket and folded it. I took out a face cloth and folded that, too. My arms felt so weak and tired, the weight of the towels made my entire body feel bogged down.

I collapsed on the couch and closed my eyes. After nearly two hours and three separate attempts, the small load of laundry that taunted me was folded and placed carefully back into its basket. With an appropriate sigh of exhaustion, I took a long nap to recover.

I forced myself to walk around every day, but eventually I couldn't even stand. As my balance faded my family and I realized a mobility aid was necessary for me to walk and gain independence.

I became an eighteen-year-old pushing around my grandma's old maroon rollator, resting on the seat when it became too hard. This fact bothered me only slightly. Once I realized how much more supported my rollator made me feel, I couldn't imagine my life without it. I was now able to retrieve my lunch and go to the bathroom alone.

As my two friends texted me about their strides of independence—from getting their driver's license to going to senior prom—I silently celebrated my milestones of standing long enough to throw a piece of luncheon meat on wheat bread.

Chapter Sixteen
Tilting Towards a Diagnosis

She desperately asked God why it was so hard to thrive
Why was she so sick and everyone else so alive?
She fought every day to get where she needed to be
There's a reason for her illness she can't yet see

— "Lifted by Others" by Shayla Rose

THE LONELY DEPRESSION coated me in a thick layer. It didn't seem to matter how hard I tried, my health would always be against me. At a time when my social life should have been bustling, it wasn't.

I didn't even know who I was anymore. I had so much time to ponder over my life, as the winter turned to spring, and summer took its place. I continued to suffer from low energy and intense symptoms.

What does God want me to be sick for? Why does He want so much to be taken away from me?

Everybody has a story. Having a debilitating, chronic illness was just a part of mine. Although I questioned the Lord's reasoning almost daily, I found comfort in knowing that His plan was greater than I could ever understand. My illness was not me—I knew that I was so much more than dizzy spells, vomiting, and intense fatigue. My illness was a part of me, though, as was the strength that my illness forced me to find.

I knew that the Lord did not wish to have anybody suffer without reason. Finding my reason for my illness became my newest search.

I dove headfirst into research and spent much of my free time using online support groups and reading websites and research articles. I was determined to know more about my illness.

A specialist named Dr. Brown was recommended to us by a family friend with high praise. He was an autonomic neurologist and appeared to have good credentials.

"Hello, I'd like to make an appointment for my daughter," my mother said with the phone pressed firmly against her ear.

After forwarding my information, my mother hung up.

"You have a tilt table test in June," my mother said as she placed the cordless phone on the wooden kitchen table.

I was both excited and nervous to hear that I would receive a tilt table test. It was a test that most doctors use to diagnose POTS—a test I had read about dozens of times. Somehow though, through all my dark days of symptoms, not one doctor had recommended this test for me. I felt that my faint cries for help were finally becoming heard.

Although the test was ordered by the office of Dr. Brown, I was not given an appointment with him. My mother called his office nearly every day, but his receptionist repetitively declined our desperate attempts to make an appointment. She made it clear I needed a diagnosis *before* seeing Dr. Brown, and even then, she would call me with an appointment. As expected, this call never came.

I stood in the middle of a bustling city. I gripped the handles of my rollator tightly and followed my parent's directions. I entered a large hospital, followed down several hallways and sat nervously in a waiting room overlooking roads and buildings.

"I'm so dizzy," I whispered to my dad as he sat at my right side, "I just want a drink!" I continued, a wrinkle forming in the center of my pale forehead.

The tilt table instructions that I received in the mail informed me not to eat or drink prior to the test. This was torture for me, as I battled chronic dehydration and hypoglycemia. Slowly, I felt like my body was giving out to thirst. First my mouth dried, my palms sweated, and my vision blurred as I followed down every symptomatic rung of the ladder to doom.

"Hi, I'm Ken!" a man with a small build and black hair turned the corner and shook my hand. "Right this way!" he escorted me down the hall and through several offices before settling into a very small room.

The room was no larger than a decent-sized bathroom, and the air was stale and stuffy. My palms continued to sweat, and my brain struggled to process Ken's instructions. As my body suffered the consequences from heat and lack of hydration, I wondered if it would be socially acceptable for me to reset the nearby thermostat. My heart raced as I looked desperately for a tiny drop of water.

"Is it okay if I take a sip of water?" I asked Ken as I held my full water bottle in my hands.

"Yes, but only a little," he insisted.

I pressed the plastic water bottle to my lips and felt the flood gates open. The water coated my sandy tongue and splashed through my throat like a refreshing wave. My body craved more—I depended on it for relief. I knew though, that anymore hydration had the potential to affect my test. It took all the self-control within me to stop at one sip, screw the cap back on, and reluctantly hand my water bottle back over to my mom.

I let out a deep sigh as I sat on the table. Ken prepared me for the test by first taping my finger to a wire.

"Don't be surprised if it turns blue," he said to me through his thick accent, "Is your heart rate always high?"

"Sometimes," I said, out of breath as I peered down at my fitness tracker. My heart rate was 120bpm as I sat there on the table, resting.

"This is electricity," Ken told me while holding a small device in his right hand.

I looked at my mother before looking back at the device as though it was a taser.

"Is that going to hurt?" I gulped.

"No," he said with a sincere chuckle, "just—just a little."

With my nerves creeping up my throat, he placed the device on my ankle.

"One... two... three!" he counted.

A tingling sensation surged through my foot and quickly went away. He repeated this electric surge several more times on various parts of my body.

"This is to test your breathing," Ken held a tube in his hand connected to a meter, "When I tell you, blow inside of this tube and try to get that meter past this line." Ken pointed to the glass meter that hovered just above my bed.

I looked at my pulsating finger. Sure enough, it was now blue. I laid on the bed thinking of how long it would take for my finger to fall off completely while Ken checked my vitals on the computer.

"Okay, now!" Ken shouted.

I blew as hard as I could, until no air remained — then, I blew even harder.

The meter barely budged. I tried again and again, until finally Ken laughed.

"That's okay," he said as I passed him the tube and attempted to smile through my flushing face. My vision pulsated, I was so out of breath, and I could barely even feel my body.

After a quick break to catch my breath, it was time for the most symptom provoking part of the entire test to begin. Ken strapped my body snug to the table with familiar, large Velcro straps. He held a remote in his hand.

Ever so carefully, the mechanical table beneath me tilted my body straight up. It seemed manageable at first, until I surpassed a certain angle and the symptoms all hit me at once.

I became so out of breath as my heart rate escalated. My vision blurred even more, and depersonalization left me in a thick

151

fog. I felt increasingly like passing out as lightheadedness overtook me and my body weakened. Having very little water in my body made my symptoms so much worse. Fainting was a sincere concern of mine as my body went haywire.

I defenselessly stood there, hovered above the floor, with my body weight supported by thick Velcro straps. My symptoms were so intense. I looked at Ken through a squinted eye as he watched the nearby clock.

"How do you feel?" he asked, looking at me worriedly.

"Like passing out. Really bad," I responded.

"Not good? We can stop," he said compassionately while watching the second hand on the clock.

He lowered the table back down to a horizontal position and unstrapped my body.

I felt like a failure and — despite the train of symptoms that my body was just struck by — I continued to blame myself. I was only tilted vertically for one minute before the test was terminated. I was supposed to stay vertical for ten minutes.

So many thoughts and emotions went through my head as I now laid horizontal and waited for Ken's next instruction.

"In a minute you need to get up really fast!" Ken told me as he waited for my body to acclimate to its new position, "When I tell you to, okay?"

We watched the clock for several minutes until finally he gave me the cue.

"Okay!" he said as he helped me stand up, "Stay still!"

He held his hands out to my sides as I stood up and he watched me struggle to find balance.

"No moving, okay?" Ken told me as I shifted my weight from one leg to the other—a common subconscious activity that many with dysautonomia do to compensate for blood pooling.

It took so much out of me to stand still, without the slightest movement in my legs.

After actively standing for several minutes, the test was complete. I excitedly left the small, stuffy room and thanked Ken for his time.

"How'd you do?" my dad asked me as we walked through the parking garage and attempted to find our car.

"Not good, I stopped the test early," I reluctantly responded.

"Shay! That's not good!" he muttered.

I hung my head in disappointment. I wished I hadn't stopped the test so soon, but I knew I couldn't possibly have continued.

We mulled over the tilt table test for the next few weeks until a packet arrived in the mail. Inside of a manila paper envelope were pages and pages of medical terms. I dissected every word until I felt confident with my interpretation.

The criteria one must meet to be diagnosed with Postural Orthostatic Tachycardia Syndrome is defined as an increase in heart rate of thirty beats per minute or more from lying to standing.

My heart rate increased by sixty-two beats during my tilt table test. So—from the looks of the papers in my hands—my diagnosis of POTS was confirmed.

Chapter Seventeen
Welcome to Adulthood, We've Been Waiting for You

The highway catches my littered thoughts
Collected with others, forgotten then sought
Automobiles double date before losing their place
Some seen again, in this city-seeking race

— *"City Bound" by Shayla Rose*

I HELD ON TO my tilt table results as if they were gold. I finally found the evidence I needed to support my claim. I was sick, and—although many people throughout my life chose to not believe that—this tilt table test showed the truth. The stack of papers in my hands finally gave others a glimpse inside of my body's wacky autonomic nervous system.

After realizing that the likelihood of being granted an appointment with Dr. Brown was almost as slim as winning the lottery, my mother and I decided to move on. We made an appointment with a new autonomic neurologist, one who was mentioned to us briefly by my tilt table technician, Ken. This new autonomic neurologist worked under Dr. Brown, whom we had originally hoped to see.

It was a spring day when the calendar laid on my mom's lap and she nervously clicked the pen gripped in her hand. The blank piece of paper that rested on the armrest of the couch soon became coated in dozens of inked flowers as my mom patiently waited for the receptionist to answer.

"You go in September," my mom stated as she hung up the phone, "so you go on your birthday, but that's okay."

I shook my head repeatedly before tensing in anger.

"Mom!" I shouted disappointedly, "That's not fair!"

Doctor appointments were always so stressful. So much of my life was consumed by my illness, and I hated to have to spend my nineteenth birthday in the office of a new doctor inside a giant city. But I had no other options.

"Can't we reschedule?" I asked my mother in frustration.

"If you don't go in September then you have to wait until April, Shayla!"

April was nearly a year away, and there was no way I could wait that long. By some stroke of luck, the doctor had an opening in September and my mom was just in time to take it.

I eventually came to terms with having to go to a new specialist on my birthday, although I spent much of the summer mulling over how it would all unfold.

The summer was very unpleasant for me. The heat was so unbearable, I couldn't spend longer than two minutes outside. The air was so dense, I felt like I was walking into a brick wall every time I opened the backdoor. My heart and air passages became so instantly overworked in the heat that I could not even hold a conversation. I tried so hard to push through—I wanted so badly to enjoy the nice weather and frequent summer company, but it was impossible.

I had so much exhaustion that I took three naps every day. I could only stay awake for two-hour intervals before I became too exhausted to function.

Every day I felt like I had pulled an all-nighter and then worked an entire shift on a fishing boat while having the flu. My limbs ached, my mind was foggy, and my heart raced.

Inevitably, during this energy depleted summer, I became depressed. I recall sitting in my backyard alongside my mom on one late morning. My head pounded in pain, my body ached in fatigue. It was time for my second nap, even though it wasn't even lunch time yet.

"I just want to be with Grandma. It seems like it would be so much easier sometimes," I told my mom through my breathless voice.

My heart was so fast, and my entire system was overworked. My grandma had passed away only a year prior, and although I didn't want to die, I knew no difference between the life I was living and the lack of life I would be living through death.

I was on the sidelines of life, I was not in the game anymore.

After sleeping through more than half of the summer, the calendar flipped to September and I was in the backseat of our car headed to the city.

Following a long car ride, I sat on the seat of my rollator inside of an elevator as my parents pressed the ninth button. A man with a husky build stood in the elevator with us. I could feel his friendly glances as my face went from a calm smile to a frightened pallor.

The elevator doors opened, and I very quickly felt faint. The hallway outside of the elevator looked as though it was moving up and down. My head began to fall as I struggled to compensate for the violent elevator drop.

"I feel like passing out!" I told my parents sternly as my dad rushed me out of the elevator, using my rollator as a wheelchair.

I began to tear up.

Why was this elevator ride so provoking?

Inside I felt like I was jumping on a trampoline, when really, I was just sitting still on my maroon rollator in the middle of a deserted hallway.

After several minutes of elevating my legs, my vertigo faded, and I regained my composure. My parents and I signed in to my neurology appointment and found our seats in the large waiting room. A television hung from the ceiling and an afternoon cooking show played on its screen. I elevated my legs on the seat of my rollator and drank my warm juice box.

After waiting a short while, the doctor walked through the waiting room and greeted me.

"Hello, nice to meet you. I'm Dr. White," she said as she reached out and shook my hand.

"Hi I'm Shayla."

"Do you want me to go in with you?" my dad asked me as I slowly stood up.

"Yes!" I said quickly, eager to receive his support and wisdom during this important doctor's appointment.

I pushed my rollator down long hallways before taking a turn into a small exam room.

I sat down in a chair right beside Dr. White's desk and I looked at her, waiting for her list of questions.

"So, tell me what's been going on."

"Okay, well I have been sick since I was thirteen and..."

I gave her an overview of my past and current symptoms. I told her about how much my illness debilitated me as she clicked away on her keyboard and nodded her head.

"These are all of the times I've thrown up. I throw up every few weeks," I told Dr. White as I passed her a small piece of wrinkled notepaper, "Why do you think I throw up? Do you think I could have cyclic vomiting syndrome?"

Dr. White shrugged her shoulders and gave me a long-winded answer, but ultimately, she couldn't tell me why I vomited so often.

"Cyclic vomiting syndrome is diagnosed through a process of elimination. You are kind of old to have it, it usually only affects children," she said in part.

I didn't believe her explanation for a second, and the way she brushed off my vomiting fits bothered me. Every few weeks I was slumped over a bucket in the middle of the night, vomiting repeatedly for hours. My fits followed a predictable pattern, but Dr. White couldn't have cared less.

"Do you check your heart rate a lot on your fitness tracker?" Dr. White asked randomly as she stared at the purple band on my left arm.

"Umm, I don't know. Sometimes I do," I replied as I glanced over at my parents.

"Do you know how off they are?" Dr. White added.

"Really? No kidding!" my dad chimed in.

"Oh yeah. They are very inaccurate, there have been studies done on it before."

"Well I mainly just wear it to track my steps," I said nervously, hoping to convince the doctor that I was not obsessing over my heart rate.

"Even that is inaccurate. Fitness trackers are notorious for being inaccurate."

I shrugged my shoulders and looked away as her confrontational tone annoyed me.

"Well come up over here," Dr. White said as she rose from her seat and walked toward the exam table.

I got up slowly, handed my water bottle to my mom and then sat down on the table where Dr. White checked my flexibility and strength.

"Well, you do have joint hypermobility," she said as she turned to grab a dull pin from a nearby drawer, "have you ever seen a geneticist?"

"Yes, a couple years ago I did," I told her as she waved for me to stand up.

I stood up and faced her as my body swayed from side to side. She used a dull pin and ran it up my leg, starting from my feet. My face changed quickly as the pin approached my sensitive thighs.

"Does this hurt?" she said, half-listening for my response.

"Yes!"

She walked back to her desk and I sat back in my chair.

"Well, you have some joint laxity, so it may be worth seeing a geneticist. How old are you?"

I turned to my parents and then I turned back to her, "I'm nineteen!" I said quickly.

"Nineteen today!" my dad spoke excitedly as he formed a smile and reinforced my response.

"Oh, okay. Well welcome to adulthood!"

"Thank you!"

"We have been waiting for you," Dr. White said humorously.

"What do you think caused my POTS?" I asked Dr. White seriously as I swallowed and braced myself for her opinion.

"Well, you are deconditioned. Do you ever exercise?"

Instantly I got angered. The word "deconditioned" sent me into a tailspin. It was an evil word to me, one that was coated in blame.

"Well, I do the exercise bike and sometimes the treadmill. But I was so active, I really don't think I was deconditioned. I was working and everything, then I got worse. And when I was thirteen, I was active. I just woke up one morning and felt dizzy and that was it. I may be deconditioned now, as a result of my illness, but it wasn't the start."

Dr. White wouldn't budge, she was firm in her belief.

"Yeah, but you had a cold, and remember the heat, Shayla?" my mother attempted to remind me, seemingly reinforcing the very ill-informed doctor's opinion.

I reluctantly nodded my head. I did not agree, but I nodded my head anyway as the voices of those around me only grew louder.

"I think we should exercise it out of you," Dr. White began, "You should start vestibular therapy. I'm going to give you a referral today. It will likely help your balance and vertigo, but I don't expect it to help much else. Send me your latest cardiac report, maybe next time we meet we can start you on a medication called midodrine."

I nodded my head, shook her hand, and pushed my rollator out of her office. I left that day with a lap full of questions.

"So, I have POTS and Ehlers Danlos Syndrome?" I asked my parents from the backseat of our car.

"Yes," they said to me in unison.

"I think you do," my mother said.

I stared blankly out the car window, and a deep, worried wrinkle formed in my forehead. Dr. White's sarcasm bothered me. I didn't like her ignorance or her blunt humor. But still, I hoped she would be able to help me.

My nineteenth birthday was small and somewhat frustrating. I spent the entire day discussing the monster that plagued my teenage years—the monster that controlled me and forced me to miss out on my adolescence.

I couldn't help but continue to be taunted by the D word for the next few days. Deconditioned was a word that, to me, was coated in blame. The D word was a myth to me. It didn't seem possible in my mind for deconditioning to be the cause of my rapid decline, not when I was always at my most active points in my life prior to my worst episodes.

I waited six long months for my next appointment with Dr. White, and sadly enough, I waited for nothing. As I walked into her office and sat down in the exam room with my parents, I sensed a different tone. Dr. White was late to my appointment, and—although I know doctors are very busy—she seemed to have better things to do than help me with my illness.

Several times during my appointment, she repeatedly checked the clock.

"Our time is almost up for today," she muttered as soon as I sat down in her office.

Knowing that my time with Dr. White was running out before it even began, I quickly asked her what she thought my diagnosis was. I asked her what the tilt table test showed, unwilling to leave without knowing her answer.

"I believe you have a mild form of postural tachycardia. You are very symptomatic," she said in part.

I was confused by her answer. It seemed so contradicting. How could an illness be both mild, and very symptomatic?

"So, do you think I have POTS then?" I asked. The tension of the conversation was beginning to heat up.

Dr. White was quick to respond, "I do not use labels because labels have consequences."

I nearly fell out of my seat. What kind of medical provider does not label their patients with a diagnosis, especially when one is so clear?

During the silence of my shock, Dr. White decided to elaborate,

"If a person says they have POTS, it is like somebody who says they have a fever, when really they have the flu," she pointed out the window to the hospital behind me before continuing, "That hospital over there is full of patients who have postural tachycardia because they are deconditioned."

I shook my head in disagreement. Why was she comparing my debilitating, six-year-long illness to others in a hospital who were simply lightheaded from spending too much time in bed? And more importantly, if POTS is merely a symptom of something greater, why wasn't she looking at the big picture and trying to find the 'flu' to my 'fever'?

I swallowed my anger and blankly listened to her dreadful opinion.

"I am not even totally convinced that you need your fludrocortisone!"

A pit formed in my stomach. My heart pounded in disbelief.

I was outraged by Dr. White's blunt, uneducated opinion. The more she talked, the more frustrated I became. I couldn't understand how somebody could look into my eyes and tell me I did not need my medication—a medication that helped tremendously to stabilize my blood pressure and slow my unbearably high heart rate. Fludrocortisone was the only medication that helped to provide me with some sort of relief against my illness. Fludrocortisone and compression stockings literally gave me the ability to stand up.

"Looks like our time is up for today!" Dr. White said as she opened the door to the exam room and escorted me and my parents out. She handed me a small stack of papers and sent me on my way.

She reached out her hand and I reluctantly shook it. She looked at me as though she didn't know how far her ignorance stretched, as though the wounds I carried from her spoken daggers were non-existent.

I left without a follow-up appointment or a treatment plan. I was sick and seeking help, but I was ignorantly pushed away. I felt insulted, and let down, as if somebody ripped my heart out and stomped on it.

I sat in the backseat of my parent's car and watched all the city buildings zoom past me. My mind was heavy with the echoes of Dr. White's voice.

"I do not use labels because labels have consequences."

165

I wasn't sure what consequences Dr. White was so afraid of. After all, isn't it a doctor's job to diagnose their patients?

Chapter Eighteen
Vestibular Victories and Visual Veers

I fought back, unwilling to surrender
My illness continued to be my greatest contender

— *"Fighting for Freedom" by Shayla Rose*

IT WAS AN OVERCAST MORNING in late September as I sat down inside of the waiting room for my vestibular therapy appointment. Depersonalization and fatigue had me caught in their web which made it very difficult for me to concentrate.

I sat upright in a tall waiting room chair. I wanted desperately to elevate my legs to compensate for my violent waves of dizziness, but I didn't. Instead, I rested my head on my mother's shoulder and closed my eyes, hoping to find some sort of relief amongst the unpredictable waves of vertigo.

"I wonder how this will go," I whispered.

I began to drift into a daydream, and suddenly I was taken back to years prior—the last time I was ever at a physical therapy appointment.

"Go and do the bike, I'll be back in five minutes," my therapist told me as she scampered away to help other patients.

I sat on a stationary bike and nervously pedaled myself away from consciousness. My body neglected me rapidly. My body weakened, my vision pulsated, my hands puddled in sweat and my heart raced drastically. It all escalated quickly, and soon I couldn't even feel my body.

Before long, I found myself lying on a bed in a fit of detachment. My body continued to putter along internally to the rhythm of the bike, even though I had already stopped pedaling.

"I'm so dizzy!" were the only three words that would come out.

My therapist hovered over me worriedly. A pillow was tucked beneath my knees and several ice packs lined my weakened legs.

"I just don't feel good. I can't do this anymore!" I melted down into a puddle of tears.

After what seemed to be an eternity of worried stares, my therapist finally caught on to my desperate—although invisible—condition.

"I don't think we should continue. It seems to be making you worse," she said.

Nobody understood why I couldn't handle exercise—not even my physical therapist. Most had never heard of POTS before, so my intense symptoms were pushed aside, until they became impossible to suppress and I was left in a very delicate and vulnerable state.

"Shayla?" A voice echoed through the waiting room and jolted me from my daydream.

"Hi, I'm Tara," a woman with an upbeat personality shook my hand before leading me and my mother into a therapy room.

Tara slowly shut the door behind her and sat on a swiveling stool. She placed her laptop on the nearby bed, and she turned her attention to me.

"So, tell me what brings you here," she began.

"Well, I have a form of dysautonomia called POTS, Postural Orthostatic Tachycardia Syndrome. I get very dizzy and stuff. My autonomic neurologist recommended that I try vestibular therapy to see if it helps," I replied.

Tara nodded her head as she typed away on her computer.

I looked around the room, assuming that this newly acquainted medical professional that sat across from me would be like most others. I assumed that she did not know what dysautonomia was, and that the entire visit would be a waste of energy and time.

"Have you ever heard of POTS before?" my mother asked as she squinted her eyes, a sure sign of her serious curiosity.

"Yes, I have actually."

We spoke about my symptoms in detail before Tara directed me to the nearby bed.
I laid flat on my back with my head hanging off the edge of the bed. Tara cradled my dizzy head in her hands and big black goggles sat over my wide opened eyes.

"Okay, just relax," she told me as she carefully jerked my head side to side, "keep your eyes open."

Every jerk of my head felt unexpected and provoked my strong feeling of falling off a cliff. The goggles that blocked my vision were connected with wires to Tara's computer. She could see my eyes on her computer monitor, and somehow, this was important in assessing my dizziness.

After a couple of minutes, the dark, symptom-provoking goggles were removed, and I acclimated to the brightly lit exam room that surrounded me. My vestibular therapist sat back down on her stool beside me.

"I can see that you are very dizzy," she stated as she carefully put the goggles away.

She began asking more questions about my symptoms and limitations. I could tell by the questions she asked that she had a good understanding of dysautonomia and its related conditions. Not only did Tara know how to rehabilitate people with balance issues, but she showed a great deal of empathy with her patients, an empathy that often made me wonder if she had faced vestibular issues herself.

I worked with Tara for several months, as she helped me to understand more of what my body was going through. She taught me ways to help combat and cope with my symptoms through special balance, optokinetic and habituation exercises. She was one of the only people in my life who seemed to accurately understand what I felt like. It was her guidance that helped me regain many abilities I had lost.

She got me on to an exercise program specifically designed for dysautonomia patients, a program created by the Children's Hospital of Philadelphia that worked to strengthen my core and leg muscles. Strengthening my body was just as important as working my vestibular system. Through repeated sessions with my therapist, I was able to improve my balance and no longer relied on my rollator for support.

Therapy became a long commitment—one that I would have to chip away at to see positive results. After several months of meeting with Tara, my health insurance stopped paying for future visits. By that point, I was very independent with my home therapy, so I said a sad goodbye to Tara, a therapist who, in many ways, helped me reclaim my life. Keeping my mental commitment to my exercises became my biggest challenge.

I had already been sick for six years, but there was one side of my illness that I would never adapt to; the unpredictable nature of it.

I went to bed the night before Halloween. My stomach cramped up so painfully which left me flopping around in my bed as I searched for a comfortable position. Finally, after much tossing and turning, I drifted off to sleep.

A couple hours later I woke up in a confused state. My entire body was covered in goosebumps, and my arms and legs shivered fiercely. My heart pounded, and I became so out of breath. I placed my shaking hand on my chest and attempted to count the beats. Nausea overcame me soon thereafter, an occurrence that was not unusual for me after such tachycardia.

"I...d...don't f... f...feel good!" I told my mother as my teeth chattered from the chills.

I took my temperature and discovered that I was running a fever, so I popped a couple of Tylenols in my mouth and sat in my dark living room beneath a pile of blankets.

Soon, after walking back and forth to the bathroom plenty of times and somehow escaping a vomiting episode, I shut my heavy eyelids and froze myself to sleep.

By morning, my entire body ached, and my fever persisted.

"Ugh, I think I'm getting a cold," I told my mother dreadfully.

I felt so exhausted, I could hardly even think. The day dragged on as I spent much of my time whining in discomfort.

Dysautonomia and the common cold do not mix well. Every baseline symptom that I upheld was only worsened by a cold, leaving me feeling like I was lying on death's doormat over the slightest sniffle.

The doorbell rang that night.

"Trick or treat!" little children shouted as they filled my front porch, holding out bags and batting their eyes for candy.

I was so weak and sick that I wore my bathrobe to the front door. I didn't want to miss what little Halloween festivities that I had left, so I attempted to push through my heavy symptoms and pretend that I was fine.

Neighborhood parents tried to work small talk with me. I showed my dimples and smiled, but inside I was fighting my body, hoping I would not fall. My legs were like rubber, and I was so fatigued I could hardly talk. I felt so detached from the world around me.

I wondered, as I stood at my front door on Halloween night, if the neighbors would account a fainting episode as a Halloween prank. In my mind this nightmarish vision played over and over.

Soon the doorbell duties were given to my parents as I laid out on the couch, trying desperately to feel better. I fell asleep in the living room that night, but when I woke up the next morning, something unexpected happened.

I opened my eyes and looked around the living room. My eyes hurt with even the slightest movement. A large grey blob sat just off-center in my vision; I was just about blind.

"I think you should go to the doctor," my mother told me.

"No, I think it's okay," I said to her, unable to see her face.

I didn't like going to the doctor because far too often I did not feel like my complaints were taken seriously. At this point in my life, I felt like it would be easier if I just dealt with my ailments at home and hoped that they went away.

Despite not wanting to go, my vision loss ultimately ruled, and my mother made an appointment with my primary care doctor. Unfortunately, she wasn't in, so a nurse practitioner took her place.

"Can you read this?" a young nurse stood down the hall on the right side of an eye chart.

"T, O, Z..." I started reading, "I can't see you," I told the woman as she pointed out which lines to read.

Soon, I sat back in the exam room, having failed an eye test for the first time in my life. After examining me, the nurse practitioner showed concern,

"I think you need to go to the emergency room," she said, "there is obviously something wrong with your vision if you can't see the woman doing the eye test."

I hung my head down in disappointment.

"Do I have to?" I begged, hoping she would say no.

"I would. I don't feel comfortable letting you go home like this. You could have meningitis," she replied, with a great deal of seriousness in her tone.

After much back and forth, I listened to the advice given to me by the nurse practitioner. I walked through the doors of the local hospital alongside my mom. After a short wait, the triage nurse showed me an eye chart and I failed it once more.

I was led down a couple of hallways and double-doors before being given a bed. I laid there for several minutes as I quietly listened to the murmur of those around me, many of whom were much sicker than I.

A young doctor with a good sense of humor pulled the curtain to my room and introduced himself to me and my mother. He assessed my vision the best he could before ordering a couple of tests.

"Great job Chicky!" the phlebotomist told me as she drew my blood and left with a full vile.

A nurse came and swabbed my nose. I gave a urine sample and then laid back in my bed quietly. After waiting a short while, the doctor returned to tell me the results.

"Your flu test came back negative and I don't think you have meningitis," he said in part.

Although the doctor was able to rule out the flu and meningitis, he was not sure what was causing my vision loss.

Due to already having POTS and Ehlers Danlos Syndrome, the doctor felt it would be important for me to have a follow-up appointment with an eye specialist. Connective tissue disorders can cause all sorts of ocular issues, so the doctor wanted to make double sure that I was okay.

I excitedly left the emergency room counting my blessings with each step.

Three eye doctors, a couple weeks, and an MRI later, I sat across from my ophthalmologist—a man with a pleasant humor and an interesting style.

The reason for my sudden visual disturbance appeared to be optic-neuritis caused by a virus. My vision improved over time and this sudden, mysterious episode seemed to be an odd fluke, one that would make me cherish my sight even more than I already had.

Chapter Nineteen
Finding My Tribe on a Lonely Bench

Inside a small white church, she heard a sound
A murmur of hope, so grand and profound

— "A Night at Church" by Shayla Rose

FOR SIX LONG YEARS I faced my illness feeling very alone. I was as isolated as ever in my fight to find my independence and health.

For a long time, I thought that I was the only one. I thought I was the only one who carried around a water bottle wherever I went. The only one who wore compression stockings under my shorts. The only one who sat on the bottom shelf at the grocery store when shopping became too hard. The only one whose medical tests came back normal, despite my intense symptoms. The only one who grieved my old life as though a part of myself died. The only one who faced such a debilitating, invisible illness. The only one—and in many ways, I was.

In my isolation I felt so many emotions, especially towards my former friends. I was jealous—angry even. Angry that they didn't ask how I was. Angry that, although they lived in the same town as me, many acted as though they never knew me. My illness was invisible, but I wasn't.

Many people did not know about the very real symptoms that I faced behind closed doors, and how hard I tried to suppress them in public. I looked good, and that was all most could see. Many did not understand that I was up all night vomiting, or that I had just spent the last hour on the couch fighting fatigue.

I cancelled plans left and right, I just couldn't keep up with others. I hated being the unreliable one, and the one who could never go out to have fun.

One day, after a short bike ride with a relative I took my helmet off and struggled to find my balance.

"Ugh, I'm so dizzy. But, hey! I did pretty good!" I told her as I placed my helmet on my handlebars.

"You could have done better," she stated, "I don't get this whole dizzy thing anyway!"

I looked down at the ground and felt myself shut down. My victories seemed so small to her, but to me they were so large. Months before I never would have been able to balance on my bike—let alone ride it.

I knew that she said these things because she just simply did not understand. How could I expect anyone to know exactly how I felt if they never faced the same struggles themselves?

It was because of this isolation and need for reassurance that I sought a support group. My diagnosis did not come with a definitive explanation or a survival guide, and I longed to find understanding. I needed my emotions, struggles and symptoms validated.

So many specialists only know dysautonomia from the outside. They base their analysis on vital signs and test results. Few know what being on the inside of dysautonomia feels like. It isn't until you are on the inside that you feel the heaviness, the entrapment and the hopelessness. I was determined to find others like me, ones who were also trapped on the inside.

A couple of times, I awoke from a deep sleep in the middle of the night with an emotional, achy throat as I dreamt of encountering others who faced the same illness as me. I was so desperate for understanding that I was searching for validation on a subconscious level.

In the cold depths of winter—in 2016—my desperate dreams finally became a reality.

"Wow, I can't belieeeeeve this!" I told my parents repeatedly through my uncontrollable smile as I stood beside them in a large parking lot.

After six years of dreaming of this moment, I was finally here. Just a door and a couple flights of stairs separated me from the reassurance and acceptance I longed for. I felt like the encounter I was about to have would change my life forever.

"I think I am going to cry," I claimed as my voice cracked with emotion.

I stopped dead in my tracks as my eyes caught a glimpse of a nearby SUV with Ehlers Danlos Syndrome doodled all over the car's windows. My parents stood a couple of feet behind me, chuckling and shaking their heads.

"It just means so much to me. I've been alone for so long," I told them through my whimpers and tears.

After somewhat gaining my composure, I walked into the building completely mute. I could not speak; any vibration of my vocal cords would've broken the dam that held my river of tears from flowing.

My parents and I followed up a couple flights of stairs and finally, after a deep, calming breath, I walked into a large conference room with Christmas decorations strung about. I was just a couple steps away from attending my very first support group.

This is it! I'm finally here.

I felt as though I was floating in an unsteady fog for so long. My ship had sailed along the desolate sea for six years. But finally, I was here. I docked on an island, in the company of the unhealthy, the ones just like me.

I signed my name on a sheet of paper and nervously introduced my dizzy self to those around me.

A pair of young women, both in their mid-twenties, sat beside each other. I watched them from across the room as they — in unison—spun two chairs around and elevated their legs. Within seconds my eyes welled up with tears. My parents handed me tissues and attempted to console me.

I never had that bond before—never did I have that mutual understanding of my illness with any other human. The two girls sitting across the room were clearly very close. Their symptoms almost seemed as in-sync as their friendship.

After my tears dried, I walked over to them. I introduced myself as I clung to my water bottle and they clung to theirs. We talked of our illnesses, how long we had faced them, and how we coped with certain symptoms. We laughed, sharing in each other's humor, and we shook our heads, sharing in each other's irreplaceable losses.

A sentence was thrown around in our conversation, one that made it all make sense.

"I found my tribe," one of the girls said.

I went home that day with a grand hope. Yes, I too, had finally found my tribe—after years of feeling misplaced.

Ever since the initial onset of my illness, I felt outcasted. I didn't belong anywhere, or to anyone. My friends were no longer my friends, and my school was no longer my school. I was lost and drifting.

Being chronically ill is like being sucked into a time-warp. Time is vacant to you. Your life seized at the very onset of your illness. The people and places that surrounded you prior to this unimaginable time-warp now become stagnant figures in your mind. Years pass by, but you are merely existing. Your mind, your soul, your healthy life, is still being held captive in the past, but you are without a time machine to retrieve it.

I laid on the old grey couch in my family's living room in exhaustion. My tablet was nearly too heavy to hold between my exhausted fingertips. I logged on to *Facebook* and was soon dragged through an unexpected tour down the road of missed opportunities.

An old picture came up on my screen of three former friends. Their faces were beaming with pride as they all clung to their diplomas. I rubbed my eyes and attempted to pick up my sunken heart.

It was hard for me to process, I wasn't sure how my friends—a group I was once a part of—had grown up so much without me. I couldn't understand why I wasn't standing with them to also experience a proper high school graduation. I couldn't process why my name was never called upon by my former high school principal when he reached out to each student. I was still a part of that class, wasn't I? Time went on, and my former friends continued without me. This fact broke my heart.

It was just after dinner time in late winter as I slipped my coat and shoes on and walked out the front door of my house. I sat in the backseat of my mother's car and I closed my eyes, attempting to refocus my mind as butterflies fluttered through my stomach. My teeth clenched, and my temples ached. I rubbed my head before begging the age-old question.

"Are we there yet?" I asked my parents.

"Almost," they replied.

Before long we were parked outside of a white church. I sipped Gatorade and I took a deep breath before walking into the faithful building with my parents. After following down a dim hallway, I found a room full of people.

"Is this the teen night?" I asked a couple of adults who stood by the doorway.

"Yes!" they said in unison.

I turned my head and glanced around the room in surprise. Games were set up everywhere.

I reached my hand out and I introduced myself to a young girl. She shook my hand firmly and handed me a name tag and raffle tickets. I followed her as she showed me the raffle prizes and then we settled down at a nearby wooden table.

Slowly more kids filtered in, and, before long I found myself in the company of many rare, chronically ill teenagers just like me.

We did not talk about typical teenage topics—in fact, not one of us even took out a cell phone. Instead, we all sat there around a small wooden table and talked. A mutual connection held us all. We were all mere strangers turned friends, weaved together with one commonality—we were sick teens looking for understanding.

We all were faced with similar struggles. Each of us, robbed prematurely of our youth. But there was something remarkable about us all. We each held a maturity, an empathy, and a character that was seemingly as rare as our diagnoses.

There were so many times in my life when I was benched by my illness and forced to be separated from my peers. During gym class, I had to sit out and watch everyone else have fun. During field trips, I had to stay back and study because I couldn't walk as far as everyone else. During school dances, I sat on my couch at home and watched pictures filter in on my phone.

While my classmates took up fun classes like home economics, or woodworking, I sat through two periods of resource room trying to catch up on schoolwork. After school, when my peers grabbed their hockey sticks and hit the field for practice, I loaded into my mom's car and dreamt of having their energy and camaraderie.

It wasn't until I sat in the middle of a teen night in a small white church that I realized I was not sitting on the sidelines alone. There were so many others sitting beside me that I had not previously seen. The bench no longer felt as cold and lonely as it once had. My life changed in this moment.

Chapter Twenty
You Are a Trailblazer

I lay here alone in agony
Unknowing what will become of me
I'm under such an entrapping, heavy hold
My grip on the world is getting cold
If I get out alive, if I can stand again
I will let it out, what I hold within
I will let my shaking voice be heard
I will express my pain in every word
I will stand to let others see
That something did become of me

— *"Me" by Shayla Rose*

I WISH I COULD end this book by saying, "I got better".
But, I haven't yet.

I live in a world of the unknown, where the ups and
downs of my illness cannot be predicted or prevented. I live in a
body that is controlled by something greater. I am driving a car
with a misfiring engine.

I seek help from others. I sit across from doctors who look
at me, puzzled. They all too often do not think I am sick—and
labeling me with POTS is something that a lot of them refrain
from doing. Many are uneducated, and unaware of this condition.
The invisibility of this illness has caused people to think that it is
imaginary, but it is not. For those whom this illness holds—it is
entrapping, suffocating, and most of all, disabling.

185

I often tell my chronically ill peers that we are trailblazers. We are among a wave of misdiagnosed, and misunderstood POTS warriors who must blaze the trail for those who follow. Being a trailblazer is not an easy task. We encounter thorns, we maneuver through rough terrain, and we sometimes must swim across rushing rivers just to get our message across. But we do it all in hopes that someday, the overgrown trail will be nothing more than a walking path, where others can easily be sent towards the treatments and the recovery they deserve.

I'm not sure how long it will take before the overgrown trail will be a smooth walking path, but I am confident that there will be a day when our illness will be believed—a day when POTS is recognized for all its debilitating dimensions.

I sometimes hear people say they wish I never got sick at all—and I cater to that thought, too. But my illness has changed me. As much as I adore the thought of being normal—and as much as I truly crave recovery, I realize that my past has sculpted me. My illness has made me more sensitive to a silenced side of our culture. It has broken me down to my most vulnerable, fragile self. But in my silent suffering, I have found my voice, and I have found and heard the voices of countless others. I am not the same person that I was before illness—and that isn't entirely a bad thing.

There have been so many times when I have lost my will to fight. Times when my chest gets hollow, and my eyes send down streams of defeated tears. I still lose my will sometimes. I surrender to the hold of my illness and sit in a pile of unwavering grief. I cry until my head feels like it is splitting in two, until my face is soaked and raw.

In the times when I feel like giving up is the only option, I must remind myself that I have a purpose—and you do too. In times when you don't think it will ever get better, please know it will. You will have another good day. You will be able to get out of bed again—you will get stronger again.

Advocating for ourselves and for others is so important. We must go on—and continue blazing trails. Spreading awareness by educating others is the most valuable tool we have. There is so much more that must be done—in the medical community and general society, for POTS to be recognized and understood. We must never give up. We must keep on, keeping on.

You are not alone in your fight. I am here alongside you, and together, there is hope.

With love, from my tachycardic heart to yours,

Shayla Rose

ACKNOWLEDGMENTS

As I laid down in my recliner at eighteen, isolated, hopeless, and unknowing what would become of me, I begged one silent question.
"What is the reason for my illness?"
God answered that question with three simple words.
"To help others."
Inspired by this realization, I followed God's answer. I used my ability to write to honestly and openly share my story. I wrote down everything I had gone through, from the very beginning of my illness to the current moment, hoping that in turn these words could help others. In the early days of my book, I was too exhausted to work on my computer, and my hands would tire too quickly if I wrote by hand. Determined to help others by my story, I placed my fingers on my keyboard, closed my exhausted eyes, and wrote from my heart. My goal of this book is to help give others hope—a hope that was given to me by the Lord. Thank you, God, for your kindness, your gentle presence, and for giving me the grace and strength to write this book.

Thank you, Mom and Dad for being my heroes, my best friends and my strongest supporters. You guys have dried my tears, made me laugh during my darkest moments, and often have been the only ones by my side when the entire world seemed against me. Thank you for caring for me in the times when I could not care for myself, and for always reminding me to never give up. Thanks for being beside me every step of the way, no matter where the road takes us, or what crazy idea I come up with next. You both mean so much to me, and my gratitude and love for you guys is beyond words.

Thank you, Mrs. K for helping me achieve my education despite my illness. Thank you for your patience during my bad days, and for lending me an ear when I all too often broke down in tears during our lessons. Your humor made lessons pass quicker and dark days seem much lighter. You are an amazing educator whom I admire deeply. I love math, I love math, I love math.

Thank you, Clara, for giving me your wisdom and support to overcome my fears and share my talents. If it wasn't for your persistence, I would have never continued to scribe my thoughts on paper.

Keep on keeping on.